Restraint of Domestic Animals

Teresa F. Sonsthagen, RVT
Department of Veterinary Science
North Dakota State University
Fargo, North Dakota 58105

Technical Editor: Thomas P. Colville, DVM, MSc
Editor: Paul W. Pratt, VMD
Illustrations: Bill Amundson, Conery Calhoon,
Brian Evans, Les Sealing, DVM
Production Manager: Elisabeth S. Stein

American Veterinary Publications, Inc.
5782 Thornwood Drive
Goleta, California 93117

Library of Congress Card Number: 90-081325
ISBN 0-939674-28-9

Printed in the United States of America

Preface

Reading this book will not make you an expert in restraint of domestic animals. My 12 years as a veterinary technician have proven that I am not. I do not believe anyone can claim to be an expert in this discipline, because animals have a unique ability to make a fool of you when you think you are an expert.

This book was written to bring together descriptions of restraint techniques published in many other sources and to provide a "how to" book. This book was also designed to teach veterinary technician students the basic restraint techniques they will use during their careers in practice. It is my hope that they will modify and adapt these basic techniques to their own situation and develop their own style of handling animals as they grow and learn in their profession.

Teresa F. Sonsthagen, RVT

Acknowledgments

I am ever grateful for the advice given to me by the veterinarian I worked for during my training days. He took me aside 2 weeks into my externship and told me I needed to ease up on my restraint techniques. It seems I was applying maximum restraint on every patient that walked in the door. I thought I was doing great; and not a single animal got away from me! But what I did not see was the anxiety I was causing the animals, their owners and this wise veterinarian. Thank you, Dr. Aafedt. It was a lesson well learned.

Special thanks to my sister, Holly Foell-Doll, who read the manuscript and tactfully pointed out where the instructions were a bit hazy.

Last but not least, I owe a great debt of thanks to Dr. Joann Colville, Dr. Tom Colville and Eloyes Hill. Their encouragement, advice and occasional prodding were deeply appreciated.

Dedication

This is for Tucker, a special Cocker Spaniel who would be here today if only the advice given in this book had been taken to heart.

Contents

1

Introduction

Why Learn Restraint Techniques?

Veterinary medicine is dedicated to the preservation of the health and well-being of animals. As in human medicine, this involves a variety of diagnostic and therapeutic procedures. But unlike human patients, our patients are not willing to have blood samples drawn and hold perfectly still for radiographs, and sometimes even resent being handled. Therefore, veterinary technicians must learn how to properly restraint their patients.

Restraint means to hold back, check or suppress action; to keep something under control or to deprive of physical freedom. Various degrees of restraint can be used to allow the veterinarian to examine and treat our patients. Restraint in its mildest form is a gentle touch and a soft voice. For example, when first meeting a patient, a soft stroke to the head and gentle hello go a long way in gaining that animal's trust.

Restraint can also involve confinement in a corral, box stall or cage that limits the animal's movement but is not as restrictive as immobilizing a portion of the animal's body, as is necessary for jugular venipuncture. Restraint in its most restrictive form can involve causing a reduction or complete loss of muscular control by use of chemicals, such as tranquilizers, sedatives and general anesthetics.

Considerations for Restraint

Some basic guidelines should be kept in mind while you are learning and performing restraint techniques on animals: What are the effects of the restraint techniques on the animals. Is the selected restraint technique safe for the people and animals involved? What technique and equipment should be used? When and where should the restraint procedure be done? Who should perform the restraint procedure?

Effects of Restraint on Animals

The goal in any restraint procedure is to minimize the effects of handling. Improper restraint can affect an animal physically or psychologically for the rest of its life. For this reason, it is our responsibility to contain our temper, use good judgment in selecting the proper restraint techniques for each individual, and apply the minimum amount of restraint necessary to complete the procedure.

Safety Considerations

Human Safety: It is important to ensure the safety of the people involved in any restraint procedure, not only from the standpoint of maintaining their health, but for economic reasons as well. Injury to veterinary personnel means loss of income for the practice, and injury to an animal owner can result in a law suit. Before you apply any restraint to an animal, 2 important questions must be considered if you are to prevent injury.

What type of animal am I dealing with? From a behavior standpoint, most species of animals behave in a predictable manner. However, individual animals have their own tolerance level for being handled and manipulated, beyond which they object to restraint. For example, one herd of cows acts pretty much like another, and you can usually treat all herds alike. However, if you remove an individual from a herd, it can become very aggressive or it may become docile and easier to handle than it was as part of the herd. Knowing the normal behavior patterns of the various domestic species gives you important information on what makes them nervous or frightened, and helps predict how they are likely to react in a particular situation.

The "herd instinct" dictates the action of the animals involved in that group. There is safety in numbers, and if an individual of the group is threatened, the rest of the group comes to its aid. For example, when you capture a kid (baby goat), its usual reaction is to cry out. The kid's cry usually prompts the rest of the flock to come to its defense. This type of behavior is common in groups of pigs, horses and dogs, as well as goats.

Not only are there differences in behavior among individual animals, but also there are often differences in the behavior exhibited by males and females of the same species. For example, females in estrus (heat) can become dangerous and aggressive. Female horses (mares) in estrus tend to develop a short temper and do not tolerate other mares around them. The danger here is getting caught between 2 mares. Intact male cattle (bulls) are very aggressive, and can be extremely dangerous during mating season. Extreme caution should be observed when handling these animals, especially dairy bulls, whose behavior tends to be unpredictable even under normal circumstances. These are not the kinds of animals that a novice should be dealing with. If you feel uncomfortable working around these animals, do not attempt to do so, for your own safety and that of the other people involved.

Female animals with young should also be approached cautiously. All mothers can be very protective if they feel their offspring are being threatened, and will defend them to the death if necessary. Depending on the species, sometimes it is best to separate the offspring from the mother before proceeding with any treatment. For example, female pigs (sows) become enraged when they hear the squeals of their piglets or even piglets that are not their own, and attempt to come to their aid. They may climb over or force their way under corral fences to get to the piglets. In other species, such as horses, young animals should be handled within the mother's sight because the mother is more worried about the physical separation than the handling. If you move a foal out of the mare's sight, both mare and foal fret vocally and may injure themselves in the attempt to be reunited.

Some animals are extremely territorial, and quickly establish and defend their territory. For example, a cat or dog that is friendly when placed into a hospital cage or run may suddenly become very aggressive when it is brought out for examination. In this case, the animal has established the cage or run as its territory and will defend it against all invaders. The solution is to remove the animal from its territory. The easiest method is to open the door and allow the animal to walk out. Most animals become more calm when removed from their territory.

The second question to consider is, *How can this animal hurt me?* Domestic animals have teeth to bite with, beaks to peck with, hooves to kick, stomp and strike with, and claws that can puncture, scratch and dig. Large animals can use their head as a battering ram; there is always a chance of being crushed by an unrestrained large animal.

Animal Safety: Most animals do not quietly submit to forceable restraint. Their resistance may prompt you to hold on a bit tighter. Your more forceful restraint may cause the animal to resist even more, eventually resulting in injury to you or the animal.

Of the various species of animals you may work with, each has a variety of restraint techniques appropriate for that species. Your job is to match those restraint techniques with the diagnostic or therapeutic procedures being performed and to the individual animal so as to prevent injury.

Some of the animals you restrain are very young, very old, sick or injured, and cannot be treated the same as healthy animals. Very young and old animals must be treated gently. The small bones of young animals and the brittle bones of old animals can be easily broken. The joints on the very young are easily dislocated. In very old animals, manipulation of joints during restraint can cause pain.

Restraint causes stress in normal, healthy animals, and is even more stressful for very young and very old animals. Very young animals should be treated gently so that their first trips to the veterinarian are not unhappy ones. Similarly, old animals should also be treated gently so that their trips to the veterinarian are not painful.

Many of the animals handled by veterinary technicians are sick or injured, and already stressed. Rough handling during restraint may delay recovery or even lead to a premature death. Because pain can precipitate shock, restraint techniques that increase pain in an injured patient may cause death. Pregnant animals are also affected by stress, and complications may arise if they are treated harshly.

After the restraint procedure is completed, the animal should be observed for signs of injury associated with restraint. Unless chemical restraint was used, no ill effects should be noted and the animal should appear as before restraint was applied.

If an individual must be removed from a group, all of the animals should be moved into an enclosure. The individual should then be singled out, quickly removed, treated and returned to the group as promptly as possible.

There are levels of social standing in most groups of animals. There will be a dominant animal, after which there are descending levels of status in the "pecking order." An animal removed from the group for too long may lose its position in the "pecking order," and may have to fight to reestablish its position. Other members of the group may drive the animal away or even kill it.

Every time you use restraint, you must consider the safety of the animal and the people involved. With some experience, you will be able to foresee problems that could develop during a procedure, and then take precautions to prevent them. While the animal safety is important, human safety must take precedence. If possible, animal owners or nonveterinary personnel should not help restrain an animal unless absolutely necessary, as any mishap could have legal repercussions.

Restraint Procedures and Equipment

It would be wonderful if our patients would cooperate and we would not have to restrain them at all. Unfortunately, physical restraint of an animal is usually unavoidable. However, restraint does not have to be painful or very stressful. Before restraint is applied, you must use good judgment in selecting the proper restraint technique. Do not routinely use a favored technique just because it always works. Consider the animal and judge what is best for that particular individual.

Animals can be hurt and become psychologically upset if restraint is overly harsh. Restraint techniques must be applied properly and in such a manner as to minimize any pain experienced by the animal. The technician must have a good working knowledge of animal anatomy, physiology and behavior to decide what restraint technique to use for a particular procedure.

Equipment: If restraint equipment is to be used during the procedure, examine the equipment and have it nearby before starting. There is nothing more aggravating or potentially dangerous than having a piece of equipment fail to function properly or break during the restraint procedure.

The most flexible instruments for restraint are your hands. The hands can soothe and calm an animal, and manipulate any part of an animal's body for examination or treatment. But your hands can also cause fractures or suffocation if used with too much force. The hands should also be considered fragile instruments because they are easily injured by animals. So you must protect your hands by learning where and how to grasp animals.

Most restraint instruments are designed for use on a particular species, and many are designed to distract the animal by applying a small amount of pain to a different area of the body than that being worked on. These instruments can cause injury if used incorrectly but are invaluable when used correctly. Uses of many of these instruments are described in later chapters.

Voice: Another important restraint "tool" is the voice. Almost every domestic animal responds to the tone of voice used by the handler. Your voice is a powerful instrument, but it can also be used to disadvantage. Fear and lack of confidence can be conveyed by your voice. Animals are very perceptive of the tone of your voice and "body language." If you are afraid of an animal, keep quiet and stand still until you can master the fear and continue without arousing the animal's suspicion.

The most common use of the voice is to let the animal know you are approaching it. Undesirable patient behavior, such as striking out or trying to get away, can result if you suddenly appear close to an animal. It is wise to begin talking to an animal long before you get close to it. Your voice can also be useful while you are actually handling an animal. When used in combination with manual restraint, quietly speaking to the animal tends to calm the animal and the owner.

Three tones of voice are useful in letting the animal know what is expected: soothing, instructional and commanding.

Soft, crooning words in a *soothing* tone of voice should be used as long as the animal is behaving itself or while you are getting acquainted. Commonly used phrases include "Hello," "Good good," "It's OK," "Hang in there" and "Almost over." Any words can be used, as long as a soothing tone is used. Be careful not to speak too quickly or with a sense of urgency, such as when an injection is about to be given. This alerts the animal that something unpleasant is about to happen.

An *instructional* tone of voice is firm and abrupt, and is used when an animal balks or refuses to do what you are asking. Examples include "Sit," "No" and "Stop." Be very firm and decisive, and use a lower pitch than the soothing tone.

A *commanding* tone of voice is the "voice of authority." It is used when you want the animal to behave and pay attention. It should be very firm and deep, and somewhat louder than the instructional tone. However, do not scream. Screaming indicates a lack of control. The same words can be used as with the instructional tone, but the inflection is different and the consonants are drawn out. For example, "Behavvvvve!" and "Enough(fffff)!"

As with all restraint, the key to success when using your voice is to be firm and consistent. Do not begin a restraint procedure by screaming at the animal and then switching to a soothing voice. These mixed signals only confuse the animal. Should the animal be afraid of you or trust you?

Drugs: Chemical restraint is the most recently developed type of restraint. It involves use of drugs whose effects range from sedation to complete immobilization. Chemical restraint can be extremely dangerous in the hands of untrained personnel. You must know what drug and dosage to give to achieve the desired effects, and how to handle the animal once the drug has been given. Administration of chemical restraint is not to be taken lightly.

Circumstances for Restraint

The ideal setting in which to apply a restraint technique is in a clean, well-lighted, air-conditioned clinic or hospital. But you must also be prepared to perform a restraint technique under less ideal conditions. To do the best job possible, several considerations should be kept in mind while planning and implementing the restraint techniques. These considerations apply to routine circumstances but also should be applied as much as possible to emergency circumstances.

Time: The best time to apply a restraint technique depends on the species of animal and the type of restraint used. If the procedure involves general anesthesia, the animal should be anesthetized early in the day so it has the remainder of the day to recover. The time of day is also a factor when physically restraining some animals. Some animals are easily handled during their resting periods. Nocturnal animals (active at night) can be handled more easily in bright light. Conversely, diurnal animals (active during the day) are handled more easily in subdued lighting.

Temperature: Hot or cold weather conditions can cause problems in restraint. Some species, such as pigs and sheep, become hyperthermic (overheated) quickly if handled roughly or chased excessively in hot weather. If possible, plan procedures that require physical restraint for cooler periods of the day. Early morning is often the best time because it is usually cool and the animals can be observed for problems the rest of the day. In emergency situations, various safety measures can help protect the animal from the adverse effects of heat. These include performing the restraint procedure in an area that will remain shady for most of the day, using fans and cool water sprayed on the animal's legs and stomach to cool it, and avoiding heavy restraint techniques when the humidity is higher than 70%.

In cold weather, hypothermia (lower than normal body temperature) is a concern when animals are to be restrained. Taking advantage of solar heat is wise if a heated barn is not available. This is especially important in animals that have been anesthetized, as their body temperature decreases under anesthesia. Animals anesthetized in a cold environment may become dangerously hypothermic.

Setting: The physical environment in which you are working also demands attention. Small animals, such as dogs, cats, rodents and birds, are usually restrained in an examination room or hospital treatment area. Doors and windows should be securely latched to prevent escape and countertops cleared of excess equipment. When large animals are to be herded into chutes or corrals, these structures should be inspected before the animals are moved into them. Check for loose boards and protruding nails or splinters. Also check mechanical equipment for proper working condition. If an animal is to be cast (laid down), the area should be cleared of objects that could cause injury.

Personnel

Both veterinarians and veterinary technicians are capable of restraining animals. The person selected to apply the restraint depends on the procedure to be done, help available and circumstances involved. For example, when I worked in a veterinary practice, one of the veterinarians would restrain the dogs while I did the cephalic venipunctures. This type of cooperative effort worked well for all concerned. For herd work in the same practice, I caught the cattle in the squeeze chute and gave the vaccinations. This freed the veterinarian to do rectal palpations and administer a dose of dewormer.

Planning

As part of the veterinary team, technicians must ensure that animals under their care are treated in the best manner possible. This means that every restraint procedure must be preceded by thorough planning to ensure the safety of everyone involved. You must know which restraint techniques work well on the various types of animals. When a combination of procedures will be used, you must plan the sequence of restraint techniques so that you can switch from one to another without having to stop and decide upon the next step. Also, the animal's temperament may change as the procedure is carried out, so you should start with the least amount of restraint possible and work into more restrictive techniques as needed.

Duration

The duration of the restraint technique must also be taken into consideration. You should not initiate a restraint technique until everyone is ready to do their part of the procedure. An animal held in an unnatural position for a prolonged period begins to struggle, making the procedure stressful for you and the animal. The restraint technique should be applied quickly and firmly. Serious injuries can result if it is applied sloppily or incorrectly. You must know how to restrain the animal before you apply any restraint. If you are unsure of how to apply a specific type of restraint, it should not be attempted.

Complications

Regardless of how well a restraint technique is planned, unpredicted events may cause problems. By anticipating problems, you can better deal with them if and when they occur. Some animals do not respond to gentle words and caresses. In such cases, drastic measures must be taken to control these animals. The main point to remember in these situations is not to lose your temper. If you become angry, you decrease the likelihood that the animal will cooperate.

As you review the following chapters, bear in mind that you must always strive to use the minimum amount of restraint necessary to complete a procedure. This does not mean that you should apply *no* restraint, as that could result in injury.

Rather, begin with a gentle hand and a reassuring voice, then progressively apply more restraint as needed.

References

1. Fowler ME: *Restraint and Handling of Wild and Domestic Animals*. Iowa State Univ Press, Ames, 1978. pp 3-16.

2. Leahy JR and Barrow P: *Restraint of Animals*. Cornell Campus Store, Ithaca, NY, 1953.

3. Neil DH and Kessel ML, in McCurnin D: *Clinical Textbook for Veterinary Technicians*. Saunders, Philadelphia, 1986.

2

Knot Tying

Often the restraint of large animals requires use of ropes and knots to secure them to objects or to immobilize them. It is therefore important that you learn how to tie the basic knots and hitches used in restraining animals.

Terminology[1-4]

Knots are an "intertwining of one or two ropes in which the pressure of the standing part of the rope alone prevents the end from slipping."[2]

Hitches are a "temporary fastening of a rope to a hook, post or other object, with the rope arranged so that the standing part forces the end against the object with sufficient pressure to prevent slipping."[2]

The *standing part* of the rope is the longer end of the rope or the end attached to the animal.

The *end* is the short end of the rope or the end that can be freely moved about.

A *bight* is a sharp bend in the rope.

A *loop or half hitch* is a complete circle formed in the rope. A loop can open toward you or away from you (Fig 1). Careful attention to how a loop is made ensures that your knots or hitches will be successful.

Figure 1. A loop or half hitch. A. Opening   Figure 2. Overhand knot.
toward you. B. Opening away from you.

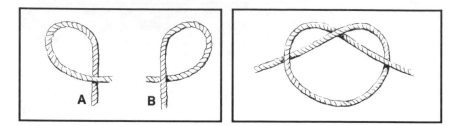

A *throw* is when one rope is wrapped around another to make part of a knot.

An *overhand knot* is the base knot for a number of different knots (Fig 2). It is made by making a half hitch and then bringing the end through the resulting loop.

Equipment Maintenance[2]

It is important to inspect the ropes being used for tears or stressed points in their strands, dirt and kinks. All of these weaken the rope, causing it to give way under stress. If the rope is soiled, wash it in warm water. Avoid using detergents or soaps, as they can cause deterioration of the rope's fibers, weakening the rope. After the rope is cleaned, allow it to dry thoroughly before putting it away so that it does not become moldy.

Ropes being stored should be properly coiled or secured to prevent kinks or twists. "Hanking" is one method that works very well on long lengths of rope and electrical cords. Start by making a loop that opens toward you at one end of the rope. Hold the loop in place with your left hand. With your right hand, reach through the loop and grasp the standing portion of the rope and pull a bight through the loop. This bight now becomes the next loop. Continue in this manner until the rope is "chain crocheted" to the opposite end. To fasten the rope after reaching the opposite end, simply pass the end through the last loop made and tighten it. To unravel the rope, remove the end from the last loop made and pull; it should unravel easily. If not, you probably have the wrong end.

Figure 3. Whipping.

Whipping

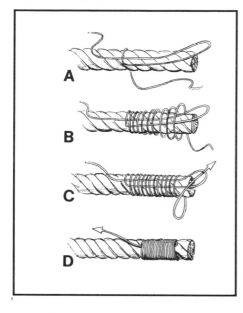

Figure 3. Whipping.

Another important part of maintaining equipment is to prevent unraveling or fraying of the ends of the rope. The 3 easiest methods are with a simple overhand knot on the ends, melting the ends (nylon ropes), and whipping. Whipping is done with a smaller-diameter cord than the rope being whipped. Begin about 1-1 1/2 inches away from the end of the rope, so as to prevent the whipping from falling off the end. Lay about 4 inches of the smaller cord lengthwise near the tip of the rope. Make a bight close to the end of the rope, with the smaller cord running down so you have 2 strands 4 inches long (Fig 3A). Start to wrap the cord around the 2 strands and the rope, making sure to leave a small tag below the wrapped strands (Fig 3B). Once you have covered both strands of the cord completely, bring the end of the cord through the bight (Fig 3C). The last step is to bury the bight with the end under the wrapped strands of rope. This is done by pulling on the tag left uncovered (Fig 3D). Clip the tag off close to the wrap to finish the whipping process.

Types of Knots

Square Knot

The square knot is used to secure the ends of 2 ropes together or to form a nonslipping noose. A nonslip knot is one that will not come untied or tighten if pressure is applied to both ends. An easy way to remember how to tie a square knot is to use the saying "right over left, left over right" (Fig 4). The same rope used to make the first throw should be used to make the second. A properly tied square knot forms what looks like 2 intertwined loops and is easily untied when the opposite ends are pushed together (Fig 4).

Surgeon's Knot

The surgeon's knot starts with 2 throws on the first half of the knot (Fig 5). This keeps the knot from slipping while a square knot is placed on top of the throw. As in the square knot, it is important to use the same end that made the first throw to continue making the next 2. The surgeon's knot should always have a square knot on top to keep it secure.

Reefer's Knot
(Single Bow Knot)

The reefer's knot is the same as the square knot, with one exception. The second throw is made by first forming a bight in the left-hand rope and tightening the knot with the bight in place (Fig 6). Be sure to use the correct rope to form a square knot. To tighten this knot, pull the middle of the bight in one direction and the ends in the opposite direction. Pulling on the end of the bight creates a quick-release square knot.

Figure 4. Square knot. The rope used to make the first throw should also be used to make the second.

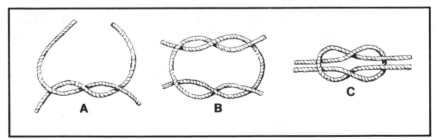

Figure 5. A. Surgeon's knot. B. A square knot must be placed on top of the surgeon's knot to make it stable.

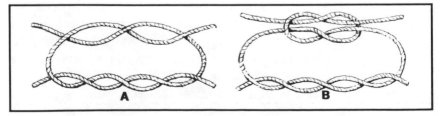

Figure 6. The reefer's knot or single bow knot is a quick-release square knot.

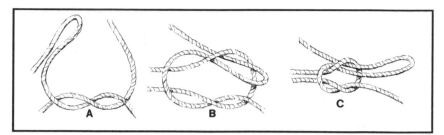

Tomfool Knot
(Double Bow Knot)

The tomfool knot is another variation of the square knot that is used to bind 2 limbs together. To make the tomfool knot, find the center of the rope, make a loop so that it opens toward you, and hold the loop in your left hand. Make a second loop that opens away from you and hold it in your right hand (Fig 7A). Move the 2 loops so the right one is underneath and half way across the left. Wrap your index finger around the side of the left-hand loop as your index and middle fingers grasp the side of the right-hand loop. Slide the right side up through the left loop, and the left side down through the right loop (Fig 7B). The result is 2 adjustable loops that open when you pull on the loops themselves and close when you pull on the ends (Fig 7C). A properly tied tomfool knot is easily untied by pulling on the ends of the rope. To secure the knot more firmly, place a square knot or reefer's knot on top of the resulting knot to hold the loops at the desired size.

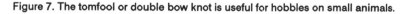

Figure 7. The tomfool or double bow knot is useful for hobbles on small animals.

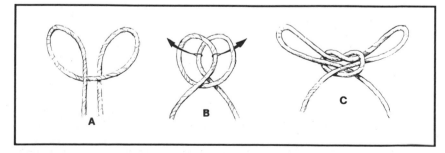

Halter Tie or Quick-Release Knot

The halter tie is a quick-release knot that should always be used when securing an animal to an immovable object. If the animal becomes entangled in the rope, is frightened or goes down for any reason, a quick pull on the end of the rope releases the animal so that it is not injured while struggling. Once you learn the basic knot, practice using it on a real horse or cow attached to the standing part of your rope, or have someone hold the standing part.

To tie the halter knot, pass the end of the rope around the post or rail, and make a loop in it that opens toward you, fairly close to the post (Fig 8A). Lay the loop on top of the standing part of the rope, holding onto the loop and the standing part with your left hand. Make a bight slightly farther down on the end, and pass it behind the standing part of the rope and up through the loop. (Figs 8B,8C). Pull only the bight through the loop, leaving the protruding end to be used to loosen the knot. To be sure it is a quick-release knot, pull on the end of the rope; the knot should come untied without any resistance (Fig 8D).

When tying an animal to an immovable object, always keep the rope short enough and high enough so the animal cannot step over the rope or become entangled in it. To keep an animal from releasing itself by pulling on the end, put the end through the loop. Note that the end must be pulled back out of the loop to release the knot.

Figure 8. A halter tie or quick-release knot is used to tie an animal to an immovable object.

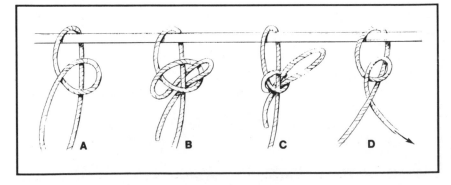

Sheet Bend

The sheet bend is used to tie 2 ropes of different sizes securely together. Make a bight in the larger rope and run the end of the smaller rope through the center of the bight, then back around behind the 2 parts of the bight in the larger rope (Fig 9A). Bring it under the smaller cord (Fig 9B) and tighten by pulling on the end of the smaller cord (Fig 9C).

This knot can be used as a tail tie on a horse or cow. When using it on the tail, be sure the rope is applied beyond the last coccygeal vertebra. When tightening the knot, pull on the end until the knot is closed, then use the standing part to tighten it. Pulling only on the end allows the knot to slip off the tail.

Bowline

There are many variations of the bowline knot. The principle is to make a nonslip noose that will not tighten. The resulting noose is safe to place around an animal's neck and easy to untie. To start the knot, make a loop so that it opens away from you in the standing part of the rope (Fig 10A). Bring the end of the rope through the loop from the back (Fig 10B), then pass the end around the standing part of the rope

Figure 9. The sheet bend is a good knot for tying 2 different sizes of ropes together.

Figure 10. The bowline knot provides a nonslip noose.

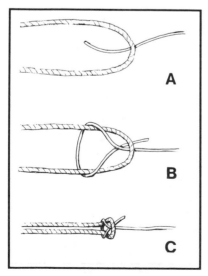

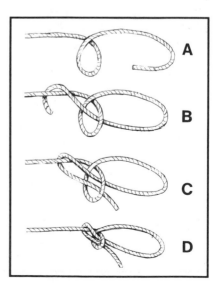

and back through the loop, this time from the front (Fig 10C). The knot is tightened by drawing the end upward and the standing part downward (Fig 10D).

The following saying can help you remember how to tie this knot. The end of the rope is referred to as the rabbit and the standing part is referred to as the tree. After making the loop, "the rabbit comes out of its hole, goes around behind the tree, and back into its hole."

Bowline on the Bight

This is a good knot for placing a rope around a horse's or cow's neck when the ends must be free and of equal length. The knot does not tighten because it is a bowline; it is also easy to untie. Double the rope in half and make a loop that opens toward you (Fig 11A). Tie an overhand knot, leaving a large bight (Fig 11B). Reach through the bight with your right hand and grasp the bottom of the overhand knot. With your left hand, grasp the middle of the bight and, while moving the

Figure 11. The bowline on the bight is used if a nonslip noose is needed with 2 equal lengths of rope that are free to be tied onto the animal. A. Divide the rope in half. B. Form an overhand knot. C. Left hand brings bight toward the end of the rope(a). Right hand reaches through the bight and grasps the loop (b).D. Using both hands, pull the knot tight. E. Finished knot.

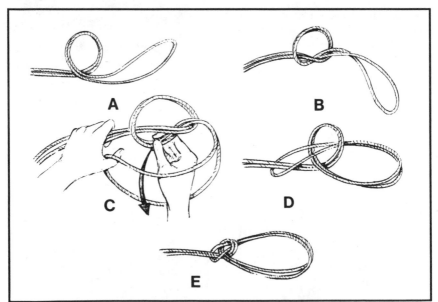

right hand back and up, pull the bight to the left until the right hand is all the way through the bight (Fig 11C). Release the bight with the left hand but continue to hold onto the loop with the right hand. With both hands, pull the 2 sides of the loop in opposite directions to tighten the knot (Fig 11D). If you slide the knot down to the bight instead of pulling on both sides of the loop, the resulting knot is a sliding noose that is very dangerous around an animal's neck (Fig 11E).

Half Hitch

The half hitch is a loop that can either be opened toward or away from you, depending on the requirements of the knot. The half hitch is good as a temporary fastening if steady pressure is going to be applied to the rope. It is made by passing the rope around a post or fence (Fig 12A), with the next pass going around and through the resulting loop in the standing part (Fig 12B). Pulling up on the end pinches the hitch between the standing part of the rope and the post.

Clove Hitch

The clove hitch, which is the same as 2 half hitches, is the fastest, easiest and most convenient way to secure a rope to a vertical bar. It can be used in the middle of the rope or at the ends. Tension can be applied to one or both ends of the rope, and the hitch will not slip.

Start the clove hitch by making a loop with the loop opening toward you, and another loop facing away from you (Fig 13A). This initial step is similar to that of the tomfool knot.

Figure 12. A. Half hitch. B. Two half hitches around a horizontal bar.

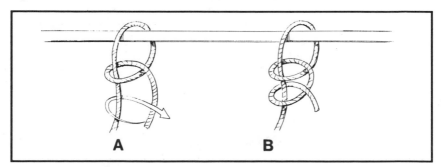

Then place both loops over the post, with the first loop made placed on first and the second directly on top of that (Fig 13B). Test each hitch's correctness by tugging on each end one at a time and then together (Fig 13C). If the knot slips, try again.

Snubbing Hitch

The snubbing hitch is used to hold an animal to a post by either a halter or nose lead (see Chapter 6 on Restraint of Cattle). It allows slack to be taken up or given and can be secured to allow the handler to perform other duties.

The snubbing hitch unsecured is simply a half hitch placed around a post or brace on a chute. To secure the hitch, simply wrap the end of the rope around the standing part 2 or more times. On the last wrap, pass the end, or make a bight (Fig 14A), between the end and the standing part (Fig 14B). Slack can be given by releasing the bight and pulling down on the end.

Figure 13. The clove hitch is the same as 2 half hitches.

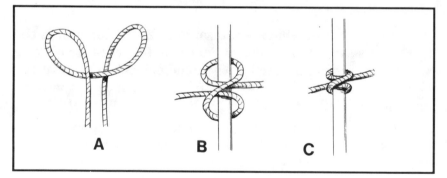

Figure 14. The snubbing hitch is used to tie nose leads or halters to chutes or stanchions.

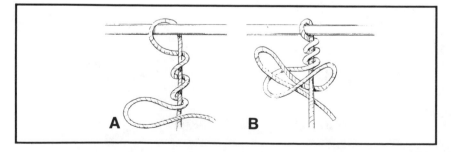

References

1. Dent GJ: *Ropework*. Extension Bulletin 192, Univ Minnesota, Agricultural Extension Service, 1964.

2. Fowler ME: *Restraint and Handling of Wild and Domestic Animals*. Iowa State Univ Press, Ames, 1978. pp 17-34.

3. Lundstrom DR: *Rope and Its Uses*. Cooperative Extension Service, North Dakota State Univ Circular A-489, 1977.

4. Leahy JR and Barrow P: *Restraint of Animals*. Cornell Campus Store, Ithaca, NY, 1953. pp 6-37.

3

Restraint of Cats

Despite our attempts to domesticate cats, they retain much of their instinctive behavior as their ancestors. Cats have always relied on their speed, agility, caution, needle-sharp teeth and dagger-like claws for survival.

One cannot establish dominance over a cat as with a dog. Cats are also very territorial and mark their territory by spraying urine or rubbing their body against posts, trees and other objects. When a cat is placed into a cage, it may stake out the litter box, establishing its own territory and defending it accordingly. Alternatively, it may become docile and rather cautious in its new environment.

Some cats will not tolerate invasion of their territory, such as when you try to remove them from their cage or physically restrain them, without some show of defense. One way to avoid provoking the defense mode is to allow the cat to meet you on its own terms. A greeting between 2 cats consists of touching noses. You can mimic this greeting by permitting the cat to sniff your extended hand. This can be your way of introducing yourself as a friendly cat. It also is helpful to talk softly and firmly stroke their backs all the way to the tailhead as you gently pick them up or maneuver them into position for restraint.

Precautions for Restraining Cats

There are some important rules to follow when handling cats. First, be sure all doors, windows and cabinets are closed because an escaped cat can squeeze through a very small opening. Remove all bottles and equipment from the countertops because they may be knocked over if the cat attempts to escape. A very important point is that each cat has a unique personality and a restraint technique that works on one cat may be totally unproductive on another. You cannot treat all cats alike when it comes to restraint, in contrast to most dogs. Above all, maintain your sense of humor. If the cat is extremely agitated, do not continue the procedure. Allow the cat to calm down, then try again with a less offensive method of restraint. It does no good to lose your temper, as this may lead to injury.

Your goal as a veterinary technician is to apply restraint to allow examination and/or treatment, and to prevent physical or psychological harm of the veterinarian, owner, yourself and the cat. Remember, with cats, apply only the minimum amount of restraint necessary to get the job done.

Guidelines for Restraining Cats

Restraining the Legs[1]

Always place an index or middle finger between the 2 legs (front or back). This provides a better grip to prevent escape.

Restraining the Head [2,5,7]

Mandible Hold: Place the palm of your hand under the cat's chin, using your fingers to firmly grasp the mandible.

Scruff of the Neck: With one hand, grasp as much of the loose skin on the back of the cat's neck as possible. This stretches the head up slightly and keeps the cat from turning its head to bite.

Fetal Hold [1,2]

You can turn the instinctive reactions of hostile or frightened cats to your advantage. When a queen believes her kittens are in danger, she moves them to safety by carrying them by the scruff of the neck. The kitten's response is to go limp, draw its hind feet up and tuck its tail up. This response persists to some degree in adult cats. If a cat begins to struggle, lift the animal off of the table by the scruff of the neck. Place your other hand on the back, and push the animal away from you. This usually allows you to put the cat into a cage or calm it down enough to resume the procedure (Fig 1). If the cat suddenly decides to jump or escape, quickly lifting the animal into the air by the scruff of the neck can again immobilize it.

Obese or very large cats are not good candidates for this method of restraint because their extreme weight can damage the muscles and skin of the back of the neck. If you must use this technique, support the animal's rear end with your free hand. Many cat owners do not understand the principle behind this type of hold, so it should generally be reserved for special cases in their presence and for hospitalized cats and others separated from their owners.

Distraction Techniques[6,8]

A cat's attention can be diverted to other things while unpleasant procedures are being performed. Talking in a soothing tone, scratching the ears or under the chin, or gently stroking the body may keep a cat's mind off of an examination or injection if used in conjunction with moderate restraint. You must be careful not to convey anxiety to the cat by increasing your strokes and urging it to "be good" just as the injection is being given or a painful examination begins. Rather, the stroking and soothing talk should continue as the procedure is performed. Be prepared to make adjustments to your restraint procedure if the cat's temperament should change.

Two other distraction techniques involve the ears. The head can be held with one hand and the base of one ear grasped with the other. A second method is to place a small rubber band around the base of both ears. This does not harm the cat in any way if the rubber band is not too tight. Once the rubber band is in place, most cats sit very still and allow you to administer oral and ophthalmic medications. After removing the rubber band, massage the base of the ears and talk soothingly to the cat.

Handling Kenneled Cats

Handling Friendly Cats[7]

Removing a cat from a cage can be tricky, especially if the cat does not want to be moved. It works well to allow the cat to come to the front of the cage voluntarily so that you can introduce yourself and make friends before attempting to remove the animal. Once the cat is at the front of the cage, reach around its body with one hand and grasp its front legs, slide the cat's body close to yours, and use your elbow to secure its body against yours. The other hand should control the cat's head with the mandible hold (Fig 2). This hold also works well for transporting the cat from one place to another. It is important to hold the front feet in the manner described so that the cat cannot twist its body and possibly claw your chest or face in an effort to escape.

Figure 1. The fetal hold. If the cat begins to struggle, place your free hand on the animal's back and push it away from you.   Figure 2. Carrying a cat.

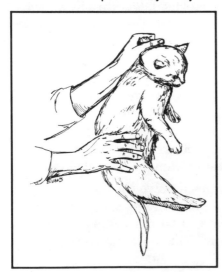
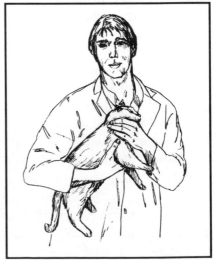

Handling Unfriendly Cats[2,7,8]

If the cat is fractious and ignores your best efforts to make friends, other options may be tried. The first involves throwing a towel or blanket over the entire cat. Once the blanket has landed, quickly scoop the cat up inside the blanket. Usually the cat immediately quiets down and you can maneuver the cat's body to get a better grip.

The second option uses a rope or nylon leash. Make a fairly large loop on the end of the leash, toss it over the cat's head and quickly close the loop down. This allows you to pull the animal to the front of the cage so you can pick it up. Sometimes, however, this does not work because the cat uses its front feet to deflect the rope. Occasionally the loop falls down around the cat's thorax or abdomen. Even if this happens, you can still pull the cat to the front of the cage and get a better hold on it.

The third option is to use a capture pole (see Fig 5, Chapter 4). This is a metal tube through which a plastic-coated rope passes to form an adjustable noose. The capture pole works on the same principle as a leash but the plastic coating stiffens the rope, making it harder for the cat to bat it away. The advantage of a capture pole is that it allows you to work at a distance from the cat. Using a towel or leash requires you to move your upper body inside the cage with the fractious cat, which can lead to injury. The capture pole must be used carefully to avoid injury to the cat, either as it struggles with the noose around its neck or if it bites the end of the pole.

The fourth option is to throw a fish net or some other kind of netting over the cat's body. Once the animal is entangled in the net, grasp a leg and the head so a sedative can be injected.

Use of Leather Gauntlets[2]

Leather gauntlets should be used when dealing with very aggressive cats. They consist of leather gloves with a long leather sleeve extending to the elbow. Though gauntlets will not protect you from bites, they can protect you from scratches. When wearing gauntlets, be particularly careful when grasping a cat, as these heavy gloves reduce your tactile awareness. This makes it difficult to tell how hard you may be squeezing the cat.

Once the animal is on a table or work surface, press it into the table using the "scrunch technique" (see Restraint for General Examination below). Shake off the glove on the hand holding the rear end, and then hold onto the scruff of the neck with that hand while shaking off the other glove. Once both gloves are off, shift your holds so that you have control over the cat, using either the New York hold (Fig 10) or the fetal hold (Fig 1).

Venipuncture Restraint Techniques[2,5-8]

Venipuncture involves passing a needle into a vein to withdraw blood or inject medication. Vessels commonly used for venipuncture in cats are the jugular vein, cephalic vein and medial saphenous (femoral) vein.

Jugular Venipuncture

The jugular vein is the vessel of choice for obtaining large amounts of blood or quickly infusing large volumes of fluids. Cats tend not to object to jugular restraint techniques as much as other venipuncture restraint techniques.

The paired jugular veins are located on the ventral part of the neck, on either side of the trachea (windpipe). Either of 2 techniques can be used to restrain a cat for jugular venipuncture. The first involves placing the cat on a table, grasping the front legs with one hand and the cat's head with the other, placing the index finger and thumb on either side of the mandible. The arm of the hand holding the head should also keep the cat up on its sternum while pressing its body against your side. Stretch the cat's front legs over the edge of the exam table and point the cat's nose up toward the ceiling (Fig 3).

The secret to successful jugular venipuncture is not to tilt the head so far vertically as to collapse the jugular vein, but enough to provide access to the vein. The back legs can be wrapped in a towel to prevent the cat from scratching.

The other method starts with the cat standing. With one hand, grasp as much of the scruff of the neck as possible. Pick

Figure 3. Restraint for jugular venipuncture.

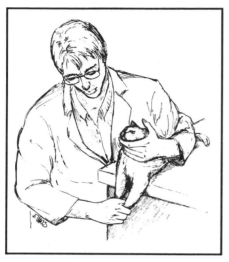

the animal up off of the table. With the other hand, grasp all 4 feet (back legs first, then the front legs) so that you can hold the front legs with your index finger placed between them. Then very swiftly but gently turn the cat over on its back. The venipuncturist then holds the cat's chin down with one hand (Fig 4).

Cephalic Venipuncture

The cephalic vein is commonly used to obtain small volumes of blood or inject small volumes of medication intravenously. It is one of the easiest veins to locate. If the vein is quickly located, the cat often does not seem to mind the restraint. The cephalic vein is located on the dorsal (cranial) surface of the forelimb, distal to (below) the elbow. To locate it, grasp the proximal (upper) forelimb and place your thumb on the dorsal surface just distal to the elbow. Support the elbow with the palm of your hand. Push the forelimb forward and occlude the vessel with your thumb, rolling it out laterally. The vessel should be visible on the midline of the dorsal surface of the leg. If it is not,

Figure 4. Jugular venipuncture restraint with the cat on its back.

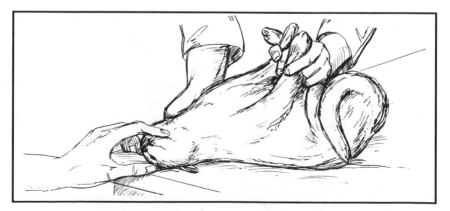

Figure 5. Restraint for cephalic venipuncture.

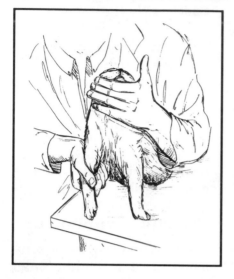

roll your thumb laterally a bit more. Support the cat's head with your other hand by reaching under the chin and grasping the mandible (Fig 5). The arm holding the leg should be around the cat's body, snuggling it up close to your body.

Femoral Venipuncture

The femoral (medial saphenous) vein is a good route for intravenous anesthesia in a fractious cat. The femoral vein is located on the medial surface of the hind limb, between the sartorius and gracilis muscles, just medial to the femur. After the cat is placed into a feline restraint bag, the handler flexes the uppermost leg into a natural position within the bag and pulls the other leg out of the bag so the venipuncturist can grasp it (Fig 6). The handler then occludes the vessel on the bottom leg, holding the uppermost leg out of the way with the same hand and holding the rest of the cat's body down with the other hand. The venipuncturist holds the distal end of the extended leg to steady it during venipuncture. The disadvantage of using this vein is that it is extremely thin walled and a hematoma can develop very easily if the needle is moved too much.

Figure 6. Cat in a restraint bag with the left hind leg in position for femoral venipuncture.

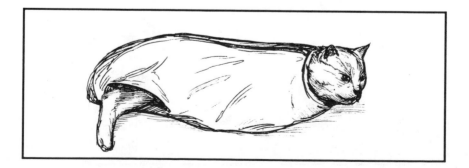

Restraint for General Examination[2,4,6]

It is often difficult to keep a cat on an exam table. The animal may want to explore the exam room, or may want to escape. One restraint technique is designed to allow the cat limited freedom during routine examinations. Place one hand under the neck, in front of the chest, and the other on top of the back near the base of the tail or around the hindquarter (Fig 7). Accompany this with soothing talk. This controls the cat's forward and backward movements without the animal feeling overly confined.

This technique is useful when the veterinarian is speaking with the client and you do not need to fully restrain the cat. It is also useful when the veterinarian wants to assess the cat's overall condition, or condition of the haircoat and skin.

Another technique involves placing one hand over the shoulders and the other over the cat's hips, and gently but firmly pushing the cat to the table. This "scrunch technique" can also be used if the cat suddenly tries to get away or claw at you. By pushing the animal straight down over its feet, it cannot easily move its feet out from under its body to scratch or run. This technique works well if the veterinarian wants to inspect the haircoat and skin or give a subcutaneous injection.

Figure 7. General table restraint technique, mainly used while taking the history and talking with the client.

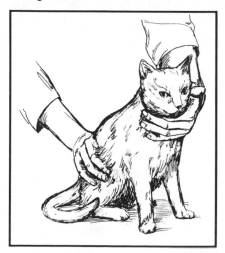

Restraint for Administering Oral, Ophthalmic and Otic Medications[1,2,6-8]

More restrictive restraint is needed to medicate or closely examine a cat's ears, eyes and mouth. Two techniques can be used to accomplish this, depending on the situation. To examine the cat's eyes, ears or mouth and

Figure 8. More restrictive restraint to allow examination or medication of the eyes, ears and mouth.

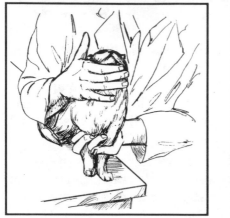

Figure 9. Restraint technique used to allow another person to manipulate the cat's head.

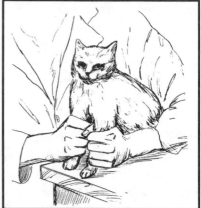

allow the veterinarian's hands to be free to maneuver require placing the cat in a sitting position. Next, back the cat into the crook of your right elbow so that the cat's back is up against your arm. Grasp the cat's head with the right hand, placing your index finger and thumb on the cat's mandible. Use your arm to snug the cat's body close to yours. The other hand should grasp the cat's front legs with the forefinger between the legs for a firmer grip (Fig 8).

With the second technique, the veterinarian or another veterinary technician can manipulate the cat's head into any position desired. Place the cat into a sitting position and back it into the crook of your elbow (Fig 9). Reach around the cat's body with your right hand and grasp the cat's right front leg. With your left hand, grasp the cat's left front leg.

Cats usually tolerate these restraint techniques as long as you talk to them and do not keep them in these positions for long periods.

Restraint for Injections[2,5-7]

A cat in lateral recumbency is lying on its side. While there are many reasons to place a cat in lateral recumbency, the most common is to give intramuscular or subcutaneous injections. Several techniques can be used to restrain a cat in lateral recumbency. The technique used depends on the circumstances.

One method is to stand the cat with its body parallel to yours. Reach over the top of the cat and, with the left hand, grasp the front legs. Grasp the back legs with the right hand. Remember to place your forefinger between the legs for a better grip. Gently and quickly lift the legs out and lay the cat's body down on the table. Once the cat is lying on the table, gently place your left forearm across the cat's neck and gently stretch the front feet in one direction and the back feet in the other. The disadvantage to this method is that some agile cats can wiggle out of this hold.

A second technique is the "New York hold," named for the student from New York who showed it to me. With the cat standing, grasp the scruff of the neck with your right hand, gathering as much loose skin as possible. Then with your left hand grasp the back legs, inserting the forefinger between the legs for a better grip. Gently lift the cat off the table. While stretching the back legs out, lay the cat on the table with its back stretched out along your right forearm (Fig 10). It is very important to stretch the cat out fully so the front legs are immobilized. Though the cat's front legs are not restrained, they are almost harmless because they can only move 1-2 inches in any direction.

Figure 10. The New York hold. Notice the restrainer has the cat's back stretched along the forearm. This is very important for proper restraint.

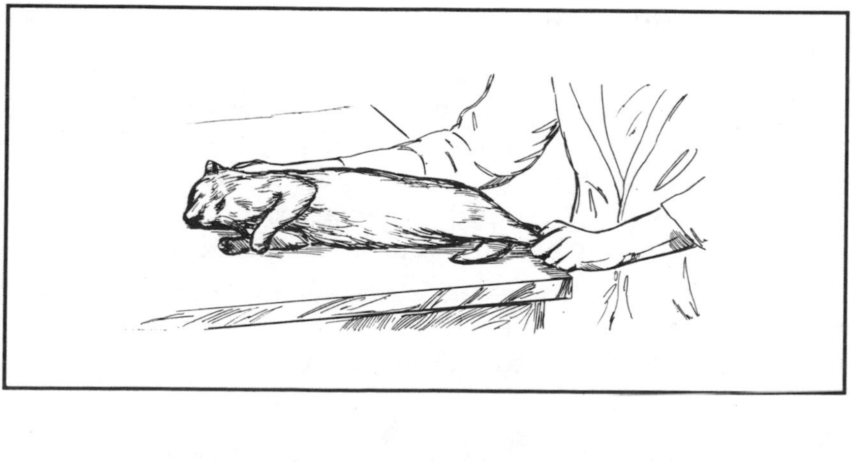

With this technique someone can give a subcutaneous injection without worrying about being scratched. This technique is also excellent for intramuscular injections because another person can grasp the uppermost hind leg or both hind legs and give the injection. Cats do not resent this technique as much as the first one described, and usually remain still for a longer period.

The last technique is much like the New York hold, but it requires 2 people. It is useful for intramuscular injection of a drug that causes pain, such as ketamine. The first person positions the cat in front of them so that its body is parallel to theirs, with the cat's head toward the left hand. With the right hand, grasp the animal's front legs. With the left hand, use a "mandible hold" or "head hold" to secure the head. The second person then grasps the back legs with the left hand. When the cat is securely held, it is gently lifted up by the legs and laid on the table. The cat should be gently stretched out as far as possible so it is in lateral recumbency with its head resting on the first handler's wrist.

Cats do not seem to mind this technique very much. I have found it very useful in giving injections with ketamine, which stings as it is injected. Once the injection is given, both people simultaneously release their holds and the cat usually rights itself and sits still.

Restraint Techniques
Requiring One Person

Restraint with Towels

A simple bath towel can be very useful for restraining cats.[2,6-8] A nervous cat can be calmed by covering its head with a towel. A towel can also be used to pick up a fractious cat by covering the entire cat and scooping the whole bundle up into your arms. You can then isolate the needed part and uncover only that area for injection or examination.

Wrapping the entire cat in a towel so only the head protrudes is called a towel wrap. Spread a large bath towel lengthwise on the exam table. Place the cat on the one-third of the towel nearest you, with its body parallel to the end of the towel. Keeping a hand on the middle of the cat's back, begin with the other (far) end of the towel and wrap it snugly around the cat. The towel should be wrapped tightly enough so the cat cannot move its legs to stand up or squirm forward. With the cat snugly wrapped, you can now examine the cat's head or pull a hind leg out for injections.

The disadvantage of the towel wrap is that with fractious cats it can be very difficult to restrain the animal long enough to get the first wrap around its body. The advantage is the same as for the feline restraint bag (see below). Once the cat is wrapped in the towel, it usually stops struggling. If the wrap is applied correctly, the cat cannot easily escape.

Restraint Bag

The feline restraint bag, otherwise known as a "cat bag," is a very useful restraint device. The fabric bag is designed "to restrict movement to a greater degree than other restraint methods and provide the handler with better protection from the cat's claws" (Fig 11).[6]

To use the restraint bag, place it on the table with the large zipper up. Lay it out as flat as possible and place the cat on top of the open bag. Bring the neck opening up and hook the bag around the cat's neck snugly. Do not apply the bag so tightly that the cat is choked, but the cat should not be able to get its head or front feet out of the neck opening. Push the cat

Figure 11. Restraint bag. A rear leg can be extracted through the bottom zipper for injections or venipuncture.

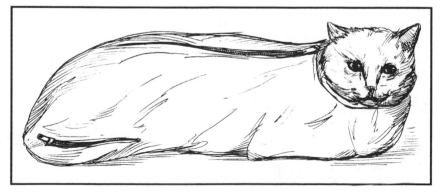

down, as in the "scrunch" hold, and zip the bag closed around the cat. *Be careful not to catch the cat's hair or skin in the zipper.* Once the cat is in the bag, it can be turned on its side and a back leg can be removed through a small zipper located on the bottom of most bags.

The main advantage of the restraint bag is that once you get the cat into it, the cat cannot escape and usually settles down. The main disadvantage is that a very angry or very obese cat is difficult if not impossible to get into the bag.

Restraint with Adhesive Tape

Taping first the back and then the front legs together is another way of immobilizing a cat.[2] Once its legs are taped, the cat usually quiets down. Light adhesive tape is better than regular bandaging tape because it does not pull out as much hair when it is removed. To remove the tape when finished with the procedure, use bandage scissors to cut the tape between the legs. Cut the front legs free first because the cat's instinct is to stand up. Its front legs will be occupied and the cat is unlikely to scratch you while you are cutting the back legs free.

"Pretzel" Hold

Veterinary technicians often must medicate a cat without assistance. This can present some problems if the procedure is painful, such as an intramuscular injection. The "pretzel" hold is very effective for restraint in such situations. Place the cat on the table with its head facing away from you. With your left hand, grasp as much skin as possible at the scruff of the neck, with your thumb to the right side of the cat's body. With your right hand, pick up the right hind leg and move it forward, hooking the hock with the thumb of your left hand (Fig 12). This grip allows you to lift the cat completely off the table so the injection can be given in the right hind leg. If you are left handed, start the technique with your right hand.

Before you attempt this technique, consider the cat's welfare. Do not keep the cat in this hold for more than 5-10 seconds because it causes discomfort. Therefore, before applying

Figure 12. The "pretzel" hold works well for giving injections when you have no assistance.

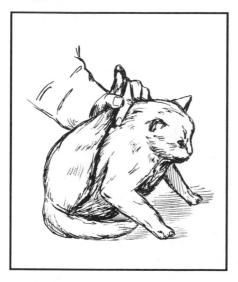

the "pretzel" hold, have the syringe filled and a cotton ball soaked in alcohol. This technique is also dangerous for obese animals, as it can strain the muscles of the neck and hind limb. Also, it is probably unwise to use this technique with a cat's owner present because it may look more painful than it actually is.

Precautions

When applying any of these single-person immobilizing techniques, *never leave the cat unattended* while in the bag, towel wrap or with the legs taped.[6] The cat could roll off of the exam table, seriously injuring itself.

Muzzles

Commercially available leather muzzles can be used on a cat, or a homemade gauze muzzle can be applied. A gauze muzzle can be made with a 2- to 3-foot length of 1-inch gauze. Place an overhand knot in the middle of the gauze to form a loop. Lower the loop over the cat's muzzle and tighten it. Bring both ends of the gauze under the jaw and tie another overhand knot beneath the mandible. Then bring both ends of the gauze up behind the ears, again tying an overhand knot. Next, take one end of the gauze down between the cat's eyes and thread it under the loops on top of the muzzle bringing the end back up between the cat's eyes and tying a bow for quick release. To remove the muzzle, untie the bow, remove the loop that passes between the eyes, and work the muzzle off with a sawing motion with the 2 long ends.

Restraining Cats with Infectious Diseases

You will at some point have to handle a cat that is infected with such contagious diseases as feline leukemia virus infection, calicivirus infection or infectious peritonitis. Some authors recommend carrying these cats by all 4 legs, extended at arms length so you do not contaminate your lab coat. This type of handling upsets the cat and may further stress a very sick cat.

A much more humane way of dealing with infectious cats is to have a separate lab coat to wear when handling cats with infectious diseases. Always treat these cats last so that you can wash the exam table off thoroughly and let it air dry for at least a half hour before placing other cats on it. Remember to always wash your hands with a germicidal soap after handling any cat, whether infectious or not.

References

1. *Medication and Force Feeding a Cat at Home. Client Information Series*. AVMA, Schaumburg, IL, 1985.

2. Fowler ME: *Restraint and Handling of Wild and Domestic Animals*. Iowa State Univ Press, Ames, 1978. pp 156-157.

3. Gilbert SG: *Pictorial Anatomy of the Cat*. Crescent Books, New York, 1984.

4. Kay D: Fraternizing with fractious felines. *Veterinary Technician* 5:190-191, 1984.

5. Leahy JR and Barrow P: *Restraint of Animals*. Cornell Campus Store, Ithaca, NY, 1953. pp 185-203.

6. Moran HC *et al*: Basic cat handling techniques. *Lab Animal* March:29-34, 1988.

7. Neil DG and Kese ML, in McCurnin DM: *Clinical Textbook for Veterinary Technicians*. Saunders, Philadelphia, 1985. pp 24-26.

8. Stansbury RL, in Catcott EJ: *Animal Health Technology*. American Veterinary Publications, Goleta, CA, 1977. pp 107-111.

9. Sayer A: *The Complete Book of the Cat*. Crescent Books, New York, 1984.

4

Restraint of Dogs

General Considerations

Most dogs brought to veterinary facilities are friendly and require minimal restraint. Despite this, it is best to be cautious with every dog. The proper way to approach an unknown dog is to extend your hand palm down, with fingers bent slightly, allowing the dog to sniff it. Watch the dog's reaction. A friendly dog's body will be relaxed, and the animal will actively sniff your hand, wag its tail and eventually lose interest in the offered hand. You can then begin gently scratching below the ear, advancing to the chest, neck, shoulders and top of the hips. A friendly dog at this point trusts you enough to allow restraint holds.

Even friendly dogs must be disciplined on occasion. When discipline is needed, keep in mind that dogs have retained some of the "pack" instincts of their wild ancestors. In wolf packs, for example, the alpha wolf (male or female) or leader of the pack keeps order by dominance over the other animals. The domestic bitch instills these same traits in her puppies in much the same way as the alpha wolf, using icy stares, low growls, direct eye contact and, if necessary, shakes and swats. We can often control unruly patients by imitating the pack leader's dominant behavior.

For example, if a patient must be reprimanded, start by looking the dog in the eye and firmly saying, "Spot, that's

41

enough!" Use a low, stern tone and draw out any "f" and "r" sounds, such as "grrrrrruff" (sounds like low growls).

If the dog does not settle down, you may have to use a physical reprimand. One technique is to grasp the skin on the sides of the neck just behind the dog's jaw. Elevate its head so you can look it in the eye and give it a quick shake, again repeating, "Enough." Do not maintain this hold for over a few seconds. If it is not immediately successful, an aggressive dog may accept the "challenge" of a direct stare and bite you. Another method is to gently "chuck" the dog under the chin with the open hand.

For any reprimand to be effective, it must be given immediately after the offense has occurred. If this timing is not strictly observed, the dog may not respond to the reprimand.

It is generally advisable not to physically reprimand a dog in front of its owner, as that can be misinterpreted as cruelty. If the dog is being unruly in the client's presence, it is best to politely ask the client to wait in the reception area or move the dog into another area of the hospital. When separated from their owners, most dogs calm down and are easier to work with because they are not "protecting" their owner. Also, the client is not there to undermine any dominance you might have gained over the dog.

A cardinal rule is *never have a client restrain their own animal*. This is important for several reasons. First, clients usually do not know the restraint techniques necessary for various procedures. The second and more important reason, is that *the veterinarian is liable if the owner is bitten*.

If the dog has behaved well during restraint, liberally praise it in "clipped, constructive tonalities".[3] Use a normal-sounding but excited voice to say, "Good dog! Well done!" Do not use a high-pitched, squeaky voice that the dog may associate with littermate sounds. This can cause the dog to think of you as an equal, which reduces your "social standing" in its eyes. Try not to go overboard with the praise; it should be short but sweet.

A trip to the veterinary clinic is, for many dogs, a traumatic experience. The different smells and the close proximity of other dogs usually causes anxiety in even the best-behaved pet. Fortunately, most dogs respond to being petted and spoken to while any type of procedure is being done. A low soft voice, gentle strokes, slow deliberate movements, and a genuine concern for the dog not only relieve the dog's fears, but also impress the dog's owner.

Potential for Injury

A dog's canine teeth can be very formidable weapons. An unfamiliar dog should always be approached with the idea that it will bite if given the chance.[4,6,7] Some breeds are notorious biters, such as Chihuahuas, Pomeranians, Poodles, Cocker Spaniels and German Shepherds. Not all individual dogs of these breeds are biters, but such reputations are usually well earned.

Special Handling

It would be wonderful if all dogs could be treated and handled the same way. However, considerations must be given to their size, shape, condition and personality. Puppies, pregnant bitches and old animals, as well as nervous, aggressive and injured dogs, all require special handling, not only for the safety of the animal but also for the safety of the handler.

Puppies: Puppies are full of energy and must be watched constantly.[4,7] They should never be placed on an exam table or countertop without having a hand always in contact with them, as they are likely to fall and injure themselves.

When procedures are performed on puppies of any breed, most sit calmly and offer no resistance. If they do squirm to try and get free, lift them up and snuggle them close to your body.

Pregnant Bitches: In the advanced stages of pregnancy, applying excessive pressure on the abdominal organs during restraint can have severe repercussions. When restraining a pregnant bitch, always be aware of where your hands are and how much pressure you are applying to the abdomen.

Old Dogs: Old dogs often are pampered pets accustomed to being treated gently.[6] Their joints are often arthritic and should not be maneuvered into awkward positions. Gentle handling is the key to working with these "old timers."

Nervous Dogs: Nervous dogs must be handled with great caution, as they can be easily provoked to bite.[4,7] A nervous dog can be recognized by shivering, an anxious expression, rapid head and ear movements, and ducking of the head. The animal may cower in a corner.

These animals often try to flee from the situation. If a cornered dog attempts to escape, never grab it as it goes by, as its instinctive reaction is to bite at the hand preventing it from reaching freedom. Some of these "fear biters" may be calmed by moving slowly, kneeling down to their level, and softly talking them out of their fears. Offer your hand for sniffing. If the dog pulls its lips back in a grimace or growls, it is best to retreat and handle it as an aggressive dog.

Aggressive Dogs: Occasionally animals do not accept your friendly advances and warn you off with a growl or some other form of body language.[1,4,7] Signs of aggression, however, may be difficult to perceive. Some dogs bite with little or no warning. Signs of impending aggression include: a head held low, either below or level with the shoulders; the gaze averted off to the side; raised hair along the back, ears down and tail straight out; and an ominous growl or snarl. Dogs showing any of these signs should be handled with extreme caution and must *always* be considered dangerous.

When you must handle an aggressive dog, 2 or more people should be involved. If one person gets into trouble, the other can help or bring help. Some handlers do not look directly at an aggressive dog, and stand sideways instead of facing the dog straight on. Both of these signals are considered "nonchallenging" in canine body language. Aggressive dogs may answer a challenge if you inadvertently issue one with your body language. If you are attacked by a dog, hold still, curl into a fetal position, raise your arm to protect your face and throat, and scream for help.

Injured Dogs: Injured dogs must always be treated with extreme caution and care.[1,4,6,7] As a rule, an injured dog should be muzzled before being moved or handled. The exception to this rule is if the injury is to the head. Care must be taken not to jar or twist broken bones when transporting these animals. The best way to transport an injured animal is on a stretcher or flat board. If none of these is available, a towel or blanket can work well, depending on the size of the animal.

To use a blanket or towel for transportation, move the animal onto the blanket by supporting all portions of its body. This may require 2 or more people to lift and shift the body. Once the animal is on the blanket, it can be moved by lifting up on the corners of the blanket. Be careful to keep the blanket as level as possible so the animal does not roll off.

Restraint Devices

Following is a list of restraint devices that can be used to help prevent injury. If used correctly and judiciously, they do not harm the animal, either physically or psychologically.

Muzzles

The 2 main types of muzzles are commercially available muzzles made of leather or wire; gauze or nylon rope muzzles you can make as needed.[1,4,6,7] Dogs can also be quickly muzzled with your bare hands.

Leather or Wire Muzzles

To be effective, leather muzzles must be fitted carefully to the dog. If a muzzle is not of the proper fit, "there may be enough play in the muzzle to allow partial opening of the mouth, and thus pinch biting" can occur.[4]

The wire muzzle, like the type used on racing Greyhounds, works well because it is designed to cover the entire muzzle. These muzzles allow the animal to pant, which allows the dog to cool itself. This is an important consideration when handling a dog on a hot day. It is always good practice to keep the muzzle on for as short a time as possible.

Gauze or Rope Muzzles

Gauze muzzles are made from a 3- to 5-foot length of roll gauze 2-3 inches wide, depending on the size of the dog. The dog should be leashed or someone should be holding the scruff or sides of the neck so the dog's head is somewhat steady. Tie a loose overhand knot in the middle of the strand of gauze to form a loop. Maneuver the loop over the dog's nose as far back as possible, and gently tighten the knot on the bridge of the nose. Next, bring the ends of the gauze beneath the mandible and tie another single overhand throw. The final step is to bring the ends of the gauze up behind the ears and tie the ends in a bow (Fig 1). If the animal starts to struggle, it can become hypoxic or may vomit. Tying the muzzle with a bow allows quick release.

A gauze or rope muzzle works well on all long-nosed breeds. Brachycephalic (short-nosed) breeds, such as Boxers or Bulldogs, require a modified muzzle to keep it on. The muzzle is placed on the dog in the same manner as previously described, except the final knot is not a bow but another single overhand throw. After that throw, take one of the ends down between the eyes and beneath the loop of gauze on top of the nose. Then bring that end back up between the eyes to the back of the neck and tie a bow (Fig 2).

To remove a gauze muzzle, untie the bow and pull the ends straight out in front of the dog so they are level with the nose. Work the ends back and forth while gently pulling. This motion pulls the muzzle off without your having to place your hands close to the dog's mouth.

Figure 1. Standard gauze muzzle.

Figure 2. Modified gauze muzzle on a short-nosed dog.

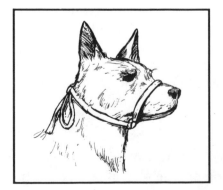

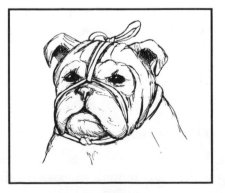

Any type of rope or cord can be used to make these types of muzzles, but the gauze muzzle is used more often because it does not slip as much and gauze is readily available. The disadvantage to gauze is that the initial loop does not stay as widely open as a loop made from rope, sometimes making it difficult to throw it over the nose of a dog that is fighting.

A word of caution: *muzzles are not foolproof.* They can slip or be pawed off, or they can stretch, allowing the dog to nip or pinch bite. Even if a dog is muzzled, check the muzzle to be sure it is properly positioned.

"Manual" Muzzles

Long-nosed and short-nosed dogs can be effectively muzzled using just your hands. One method requires only one hand, and the other uses 2 hands.

One-Handed Manual Muzzle: Place your thumb over the nose, and wrap your palm and finger down around the muzzle and mandible (Fig 3). An option is to flex your middle finger and place it between the bones of the mandible. Apply gentle pressure initially, and increase the pressure as needed. Placing the middle finger between the bones of the mandible helps prevent the head from pulling free.

Two-Handed Manual Muzzle: Place both hands on either side of the head, with your palms below the ears. Place your thumbs on the frontal bone of the skull and loop your fingers under the mandible (Fig 4). This technique works well on shorter-nosed dogs. *Be careful not to occlude the nares.*

Figure 3. One-handed "manual" muzzle.

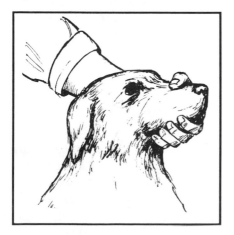

Leather Gloves

Leather gloves with gauntlets should be worn when handling vicious or aggressive dogs. The gloves do not completely protect against bites, but they can

Figure 4. Two-handed "manual" muzzle on a short-nosed dog.

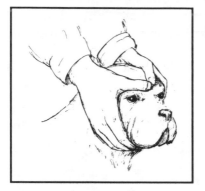

deflect "nips" and reduce the chance of serious punctures. Be aware that your sense of touch and pressure is reduced while you are wearing gloves. When working with small dogs (a high proportion of which bite), be especially aware of how tightly you are restraining them.

Rope Leashes

A rope leash is usually made of nylon rope, with a sliding noose on one end and a loop for a handle on the other.[4] It is usually used to remove dogs from a kennel or to lead dogs to another location inside or outside of the hospital.

To remove a nervous or unfriendly dog from a cage, throw the noose around the animal's neck, tighten it, and pull the dog to the front of the cage. If the cage is elevated, keep the rope taut with one hand. With the other hand, reach back and grasp one or both of the dog's back legs or support the abdomen and lower it to the floor. A large dog in a lower-level cage can be caught in the same manner, but instead of grabbing a back leg, the dog is simply led out of the cage. If the dog is extremely agitated, another leash can be applied for a cross-tying effect, or a muzzle can be placed on the dog after the first leash is applied.

Never tie a dog or any other animal to an immovable object with a rope leash and leave the animal unattended. This can easily lead to accidental strangulation.

Capture Poles

The capture pole is a long, rigid, light-weight, hollow pole with a rope or plastic-covered wire noose at its end.[4,6] One end of the noose is fastened to the pole and the other runs through the hollow pole. The noose is tightened and loosened using the free end protruding from the hollow pole (Fig 5). The pole should be long and rigid enough to support at least 100 lb.

Figure 5. Capture pole.

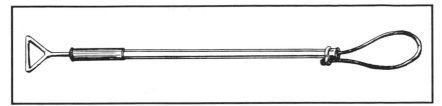

A capture pole can keep a vicious dog away from the handler's body, and controls the head enough to allow safe injection of a sedative. If the noose is too tight and begins to asphyxiate the dog, the noose is easily loosened without having to get close to the dog's head or allow the dog to escape. It can also be used to maneuver a vicious dog into a cage or run.

A word of caution about rope leashes and capture poles: *never drag a dog out of its cage and let it fall to the floor with the leash or pole around its neck.* This may fracture the dog's neck or damage the trachea and other vital structures in the neck. If the dog is very strong, 2 capture poles or a combination of a capture pole and rope leash can be used until a sedative can be injected.

Tongs

Tongs can also be used to grasp a vicious dog around the neck (Fig 6).[6] Tongs have several disadvantages. If the dog is becoming asphyxiated from an overly tight grip, the tongs cannot be loosened very much without allowing the dog to escape. Also, the handler must stand very close to the dog's body to apply the tongs, which may result in a bite. Finally, with a dog

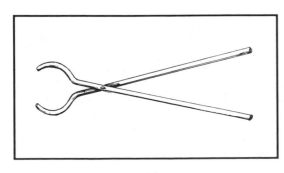

Figure 6. Tongs.

that struggles violently, the handler may close the tongs down too tightly on the dog's neck, causing injury.

Towels and Blankets

Towels and blankets work well to remove unfriendly small dogs from a cage.[4] After the towel is tossed over the dog's body, it can be scooped up and deposited onto the examination table. It is best to grasp the scruff of the neck through the towel or to wrap the towel very tightly around the dog so it cannot turn and bite your hands.

Handling Caged Dogs

Most dogs welcome the opportunity to leave their cage, and meet you at the door with tail wagging. Your main concern is to keep them from jumping to the floor and possibly injuring themselves.

The first step in removing a dog from a cage is to greet the animal. Call its name to get its attention. Never reach into the cage and touch the dog if it is sleeping. You may startle it and it may bite.

Small Dogs

In removing a small dog (under 35 lb) from a cage, call it to the front of the cage and slip your arm around the dog's trunk. Place one hand between the front legs and gently slide the dog over so that its body is facing the same way as you. Use your elbow to clamp its rear quarters against your side. With your free hand, apply a loose "manual" muzzle, with the thumb over the bridge of the nose and the fingers wrapped around the mandible (Fig 7). Lift the dog clear of the cage to transport it.

Figure 7. Carrying a small dog.

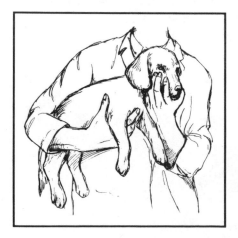

If you must carry the dog any distance, it is often easier to carry it with your arms wrapped around all 4 legs and its body held against your chest. This method allows the dog's head to be free, so a muzzle should be used if the dog is expected to bite.

Large Dogs

Larger dogs (over 35 lb) generally are kept in large cages at floor level or they may be housed in runs. A friendly dog is relatively easy to remove. Most friendly dogs meet you at the cage door, where you can slip a rope leash around the neck. They may try to slip past you, so only open the door of the cage or run to place a rope leash around the dog's neck or hook the owner's leash to the collar. The gap between the open door and side of the run or cage can be blocked with your leg. It is usually best not to use chain leashes, as they can severely injure your hand if the dog attempts to run or begins to struggle violently.

Nervous or Aggressive Dogs

Occasionally a frightened or nervous dog will not allow you to touch it or sometimes even touch the cage. In these situations it is best to try to lure the animal out of the cage with quiet, gentle urgings, standing clear of the door and allowing the dog to walk out on its own. This, of course, should only be done when the dog is in a ground-level cage. Allowing the dog out of its "territory" and into strange surroundings often calms it down. Before you allow the dog out of the cage, be sure all avenues of escape have been sealed off. Once out of the cage, the dog may try to flee. Remember not to grab at the animal with bare hands, as its natural reaction is to turn and bite.

If you cannot coax the dog out of the cage, use a capture pole or rope leash to remove it. Some dogs twist and struggle fiercely once they are captured. If you have used a rope leash, you can restrain the struggling dog by running the leash through the cage bars and snubbing its head against the door.

When the dog eventually calms down, you can call for help and use the cross-tying method already described.

For smaller dogs that refuse to move from the back of the cage, you must use the capture pole or rope leash, as described above, or grasp the animal while wearing leather gloves. Take one leather glove and place it only partially on your hand. *Do not* place your fingers all the way into the glove. Present this partially gloved hand to the dog. While it attacks that near-empty glove, the other fully gloved hand is used to grasp the dog by the scruff of the neck. Continue to distract the dog with the empty glove until you can get it to an exam table and muzzle it.

Lifting and Carrying Dogs

Before you lift any dog, consider the safety of the animal and yourself. Always talk to the dog and approach from the side, not from the front. Remember, approaching a dog from the front may constitute a challenging gesture. If the dog begins to struggle as you are picking it up, hug it closer to your chest, or set it down and start over with more comforting talk. To avoid injuring your back, always squat down and lift with your legs. Do not bend over to lift with your back. Keep the weight of the dog evenly distributed to help protect your back from strain.

Lifting and carrying small dogs were discussed in the above section on handling caged dogs (Fig 7). To lift and carry a large dog, it is advisable to have 2 people involved.

To lift the dog, the 2 people involved should squat on the same side of the dog. The person responsible for the front end should wrap one arm around the neck and the other arm under and around the chest, behind the front legs. The other person should wrap one arm around the rear end of the dog. The other arm is placed in front of the back legs, unless it is a male dog, in which case the arm should be placed directly in front of the prepuce.

When both people are positioned, they should lift simultaneously, keeping the dog as level as possible. Remember to lift with your legs and not your back, and to talk to the dog the entire time you are positioning yourselves and during lifting.

Though it is difficult to carry a large dog, the best way is to hold the dog with your arms wrapped around the front and rear legs as described in the above section on handling caged dogs. An even better method is to put the dog on a gurney (wheeled cart) and have one person steady the dog while the other person pushes the gurney.

To lift a small pregnant bitch, encircle the front and rear legs with your arms and lift. With a large bitch, it is best to have 2 people lifting, one person in front and the other in back. The person in back should be careful not to apply excessive pressure to the abdomen, spine or hips (Fig 8). Puppies should be carried by resting their chest on your forearm, with the fingers between the front legs for a surer grip. The other hand can be used to support the head under the chin or be placed on top of the neck to minimize wiggling.

General Restraint Procedures

Most dogs can be lifted onto an examination table so the veterinarian can perform whatever procedures are necessary.

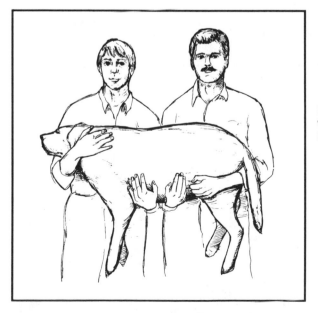

Figure 8. The proper way to carry a large pregnant bitch.

Once on the table, most dogs feel more comfortable if they are allowed to sit. Some dogs are very unstable if allowed to stand on a slippery exam table top. Allowing the dog to stand or sit depends on what procedure is to be done.

Two methods can be used to restrain a dog for most medical procedures. With the first method, the dog is sitting. If the dog is standing, place your hand on its rump and gently push down, while giving the command, "Sit." Bring the dog's body parallel to yours so you can wrap one arm around the seated hindquarters and grasp a front or back leg. Use your elbow to apply pressure to the back end of the dog to keep it sitting. The other arm is used to secure the head by wrapping it around the neck and grasping the muzzle or cradling the dog's head inside your elbow (Fig 9). This technique works well for subcutaneous injections and examination of the ears, eyes and mouth.

The position of your arms may have to be adjusted to facilitate some examinations. Dogs with pendulous ears should have the pinna (ear flap) pulled up out of the way to allow the ear to be treated or examined. You can control the front legs with one hand to prevent scratching and use the other hand to pull the ear up out of the way while holding onto the muzzle

Figure 9. Restraint technique for general examination of the head and administering medication.

Figure 10. Restraint technique for examination of the ears. In dogs with pendulous ears, the ear flap is held back by one hand.

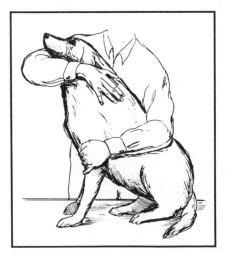

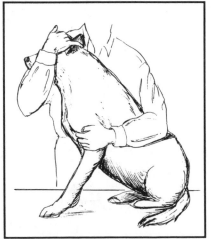

at the same time to prevent biting (Fig 10). When medicating the eyes, simply turn the head so the intended eye is toward the person administering the medication. Sometimes it is best to hold onto the head with both hands, but usually a hand around the muzzle is sufficient restraint.

When giving oral medication, the handler can elevate the head slightly and stroke the throat gently so the dog swallows all of the medication. To open the mouth, keep the dog in the same sitting position as described. Use your left hand to roll the upper lips down over the upper teeth as your right hand gently pulls the mandible down (Fig 11). Try not to allow the fingers of your left hand to move into the mouth, as you may be injured if the dog suddenly closes its mouth.

The second method is to keep the dog standing, with its body parallel to yours. One arm should encircle the dog's neck and the other arm is wrapped behind the rear quarters, or that hand can be placed between the rear legs to keep the dog standing (Fig 12). This technique can be used for general examination, and is also good for rectal examinations and intramuscular injections.

For rectal examinations, instead of placing your hands between the back legs, grasp the tail near its base and hold it up out of the way. With dogs of normal weight, you can support some of the dog's weight with the tail as long as you do not

Figure 11. Opening a dog's mouth.

Figure 12. Restraint technique used for examinations and injections with the dog standing.

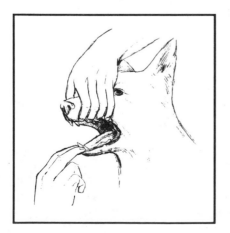

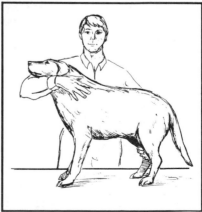

fully lift the rear by the tail. Be prepared to adjust your grasp on the tail, as the veterinarian may want to hold the tail during rectal examination. You can then support the hindquarters as mentioned above.

Bear in mind that you often must adjust your hold on the animal because of the animal's reaction to the procedures being performed. Quietly talking to the animal often helps distract it during unpleasant procedures. This also can reassure an anxious owner.

A word of caution: When the examination is over, *never allow the dog to jump from the examination table*. Most clinics have stainless-steel exam tables and tiled floors that are very slippery. The dog can injure itself if allowed to jump. Always help the animal off of the table the same way as it was put on.

Restraining Large Dogs

Dogs weighing over 75 lb can be handled more easily if left sitting or lying on the floor. For examination of the head, straddle the dog, and place one hand on either side of the head. If the animal is likely to bite, you can grasp the cheeks or the scruff of the neck. For body examinations, kneel and wrap one arm around the neck. The other arm then can be used to steady the dog or to help hold it up.

Restraining Dogs in Lateral Recumbency

In lateral recumbency, the animal is lying on its side. The basic principle is to pick up all 4 legs and let the animal slide gently to the tabletop. This can be done by yourself with small to medium-sized dogs or with a partner for large dogs.

Small to Medium-Sized Dogs

Stand the dog so its body is parallel to yours. Reach both hands over the dog and grasp both legs, front in one hand, back in the other, with a finger between them for a better grip. Gently lift the feet away from you and let the dog slide down the front of your body until the animal is lying on the table. Continue to hold the legs and pin the neck and hindquarters to the table with your forearms (Fig 13). Increase the

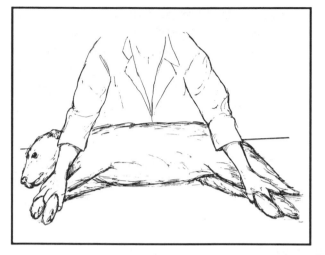

Figure 13. Dog restrained in lateral recumbency.

downward pressure on the neck and lift the legs if the dog tries to get up. If you maintain a hold on the legs that are touching the table, the dog cannot get up.

Large Dogs

The same procedure is followed for large dogs, but 2 people are usually necessary. One person handles the front legs and the other person handles the rear. Once the dog is down, one person can hold the 2 legs touching the table and apply pressure on the neck and hindquarters with the forearms.

With both large and small dogs, be careful not to exert too much pressure on the neck because you can obstruct the airway, causing the dog to panic and begin struggling.

Restraint for Venipuncture

There are 3 convenient venipuncture sites on the dog.[1,2-4,6,7] They are the jugular veins, the cephalic veins and the lateral saphenous veins. Choosing which vein to use depends on the procedure being performed. If only a small amount of blood is needed or a small amount of medication is to be injected IV, the cephalic veins work well.

If a large amount of blood is needed or a large amount of medication must be given quickly, such as IV fluids, the jugular veins are usually best. The lateral saphenous veins are usually used as "backup" veins. That is, if the other veins are not accessible, the lateral saphenous veins can be used.

During restraint for venipuncture, the technician's job involves more than keeping the animal still. You should also occlude the blood vessel proximal to (above) the venipuncture site so it stands out and can be seen, and apply gentle pressure to the venipuncture site after the needle has been withdrawn to stop bleeding.

Venipuncture can be stressful for both the animal and the venipuncturist, so it is the handler's job to calm the animal with petting and soothing words. This helps relieve the animal's anxiety.

Jugular Venipuncture

To restrain an animal for jugular venipuncture, first place the dog on a table in a sitting position, and move it to the edge of the table. From the animal's right side, reach around the opposite side of the dog with your left hand and grasp its head under the jaw or around the muzzle. With the right hand, grasp the front feet, placing a finger between the legs for a better grip, and slowly pull the legs out and over the edge of the table. Use your body to gently push the dog down so that its sternum is touching the table. At the same time, gently raise the dog's head up to expose the underside of the neck (Fig 14). Do not raise the head up too far or let it turn to either side, as this distorts the location and appearance of the

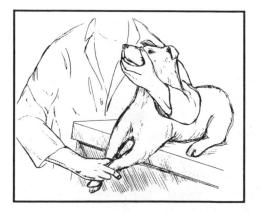

Figure 14. Restraint for jugular venipuncture.

vein. This technique works well for small dogs and dogs that object to the procedure.

With a very well-behaved medium-sized to large dog, place the dog in a sitting position, use your left hand to reach around the neck and grasp the head to elevate it, and use your right hand to keep the dog from raising its front legs. Many dogs do not seem to object to this position as much as they do to the traditional hold. This technique is not useful for small dogs because their small stature prevents maneuvering the syringe.

Cephalic Venipuncture

The cephalic vein is located on the cranial (dorsal) surface of the front leg. To restrain an animal for cephalic venipuncture, place the dog on the table in a sitting position. From the dog's right side, reach around its body with your left hand, grasp the head under the jaw or around the muzzle, and move its body close to yours for added support. Apply pressure to the dog's side with your elbow to keep it in a sitting position.

With your right hand grasp the dog's right front leg, cradling the elbow in the palm of your hand, then extend the leg by pushing it forward. Place the thumb of your right hand on top of the dog's leg, applying pressure to the vein and rotating it laterally (Fig 15). Occluding and rotating of the vein straightens it and makes it "stand out" on top of the leg. The person doing the venipuncture must steady the distal (lower) portion of the leg. If the vein cannot be entered on one leg, you

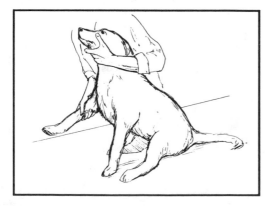

Figure 15. Restraint for cephalic venipuncture.

can switch your hold to the other leg by using your left hand to grasp the dog's left leg and your right hand to grasp the dog's muzzle.

Lateral Saphenous Venipuncture

The lateral saphenous vein is usually used when the other veins have been rendered useless or you must save the other veins for other procedures. This vein is a curved into an "S" shape and is located on the lateral surface of the hind leg just proximal to (above) the hock. The dog should be placed in lateral recumbency, with one person holding the front legs and head. Another person holds the leg that is touching the table with one hand and occludes the saphenous vein with the other (Fig 16). Grasp the rear leg in the area of the stifle (knee) joint, and apply pressure behind and squeeze the joint. At the same time, push the leg out to extend it. The person doing the venipuncture must steady the distal (lower) portion of the extended leg.

Movement-Limiting Devices

Movement-limiting devices are designed to prevent the dog's chewing on itself or bandages, or to generally restrict movement.

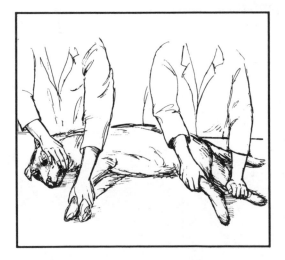

Figure 16. Restraint for lateral saphenous venipuncture.

Elizabethan Collars

Elizabethan collars are cone-shaped collars that fit around a dog's neck. They can be either attached to the dog's collar or may be just secured around the neck (Fig 17). These collars are available commercially or can be made from plastic buckets, x-ray film, cardboard (short term) or large plastic bottles. Any material can be used that is sturdy enough to withstand being knocked about or bent, thus keeping the dog from chewing or licking other areas of its body.

Some precautions must be taken when using Elizabethan collars. With a commercially available collar, the main considerations are its length and tightness. Homemade collars can present problems because many of them have sharp edges that may injure the dog's neck. With both types, you may have to show the dog how to eat with the collar in place, or elevate the food and water dishes, especially if the end of the collar extends beyond the dog's nose. Dogs also often run into walls and door frames when wearing an Elizabethan collar.

Side Braces

Side braces prevent the dog from bending its head or neck to either side. To make a side brace, measure the diameter of the base of the dog's neck. Then, in the middle of a long piece of aluminum splint rod, bend a circle of that diameter. Pad the circle well with cotton, wrap it with waterproof tape, and

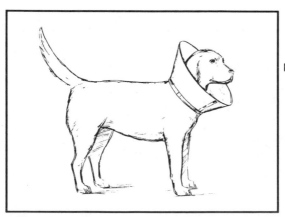

Figure 17. Elizabethan collar.

place it around the dog's neck. Next, bend the rod on each side of the circle so that they run parallel to the dog's sides. Cut the side bars off just behind the last rib. Then form a suspension band of tape over the back, connecting the end of each bar (Fig 18). Apply the tape faces together to avoid entangling the hair in the sticky side of the tape.

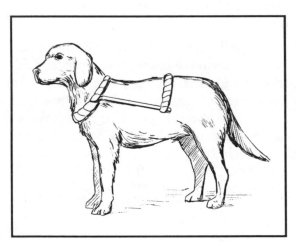

Figure 18. Side brace.

Hobbles

Hobbles can be applied to the front or back legs to restrict general activity of a dog, such as those treated for heartworm. They can be easily made with adhesive tape. Tear 2 3- to 4-foot long pieces of 2-inch adhesive tape, making one a bit shorter than the other by about 6-8 inches. Stick the tape together so the sticky sides meet, leaving 3-4 inches of exposed sticky side on each end to be used as anchors. Start with either leg by placing the tape around the metatarsus and sticking it to itself. Be sure to cover all of the exposed sticky part of the tape so that the hair does not get stuck in the hobbles. Be sure the tape is not too tight around the leg. With the other end of the tape, encircle the other metatarsus. Before anchoring the tape to the second leg, place the dog's legs in a normal standing position so the animal can walk but with difficulty (Fig 19).

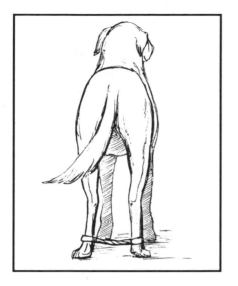

Figure 19. Tape hobbles.

References

1. Brooks DL, in Catcott EJ: *Animal Health Technology*. American Veterinary Publications, Goleta, CA, 1977. pp 98-101.

2. Crow SE and Walshaw SO: *Manual of Clinical Procedures in the Dog and Cat*. Lippincott, Philadelphia, 1987. pp 3-20.

3. Evans JM: Developing canine social skills. *Dogs U.S.A.* 3(1):64-65, 1988.

4. Fowler ME: *Restraint and Handling of Wild and Domestic Animals*. Iowa State Univ Press, Ames, 1978. pp 148-155.

5. Kazmierczak K: Bandage management in small animals. *Veterinary Technician* 3:309-315, 1982.

6. Leahy JR and Barrow P: *Restraint of Animals*. Cornell Campus Store, Ithaca, NY, 1953. pp 164-180.

7. Neil DH and Kese ML, in McCurnin DM: *Clinical Textbook for Veterinary Technicians*. Saunders, Philadelphia, 1985. pp 20-24.

5

Restraint of Horses

The size, speed, strength and personality of horses make them potentially dangerous animals to restrain. They should be treated with respect and caution, as they can severely injure or even kill you during a moment of inattentiveness. Horses are suspicious creatures, and are quick to detect nervousness in handlers. This diminishes the authority the handler may have over them. Most horses are not vicious and usually submit to properly applied restraint procedures. However, even cooperative horses can cause fatal injuries if suddenly frightened or hurt.

Horses often give some warning signals that should be heeded to prevent possible injuries. The most expressive parts of a horse are the ears. By watching their movements, you can get some impression of what the horse is feeling. An alert horse has its ears pricked forward. This shows it is aware of your approach and is curious. A nervous or uncertain horse constantly flicks its ears back and forth, especially if there is activity behind them. An angry or fearful horse often pins its ears back. Do not confuse this with the laid-back ear of a horse that is concentrating on a difficult task, such as calf roping or barrel racing.

The tail also indicates a horse's attitude. A wringing or circling tail indicates nervousness. A tail held straight down indicates pain or sleeping. A tail that is clamped tight indicates fear. Remember, each horse should be considered an individual and treated accordingly.

A horse can be calmed by an even tone of voice, and most cooperate if handled quietly and decisively. Many horses are easily "bribed" with lumps of sugar or oats. Scratching behind the ears, eye ridges and neck also help convince the horse that you mean it no harm and want to be friends.

Approaching and Capturing a Horse

Horses should be approached from the front and slightly to the left (near) side.[2-4,6,8,9] The reason for approaching from the left side is that horses are accustomed to being handled from that side. The animal may become nervous if you approach or work on the right (far) side.

As you approach the horse, watch it carefully. If it starts to move away, stop and talk to it, and maybe offer it some oats. If you keep moving toward the horse, it may think it is in danger and try to flee. Move slowly and without sudden movements, as horses are startled easily.

Once close enough to touch the animal, it is often best to scratch it behind the ears and at the base of the neck before applying a halter. After this introduction, slip the lead rope over the horse's neck and catch the end as it comes into your reach, tie a single overhand knot to keep the rope from slipping off. Most horses believe they are caught and stand peacefully, but be alert for the possibility that something may frighten the horse, causing it to bolt. If this happens, a quick hand on the rope looped around the horse's neck and some gentle talking should calm it down. If the horse panics and begins resisting restraint, it is better to let it go than to be injured trying to restrain it.

Some horses quickly learn that a rope and/or halter slung over a human's shoulder means they must go to work and will not allow you to catch them. For these horses it is best to keep the ropes hidden from view until you are up close. Baling twine or a small rope works well with these horses, as it is more easily concealed and need not be very strong; once the horse is caught, it usually submits quietly. More nervous horses must be enclosed in a smaller pen to catch them. Luring them into the pen with oats is much better than chasing them in because they are then less excited.

If all else fails, try to rope them. Again, it is better to have them in a fairly small pen for this. Keep your movements slow and deliberate. Do not swing the rope around your head like you are going to rope a calf. It is best to use a low backhand technique. Hold the rope at waist height and make a loop that just brushes the ground (Fig 1). The major portion of the rope should be coiled and held loosely in the left hand so it can peel off after the horse is caught. Hold the loop in the right hand on the left side of your body, palm facing toward you, then situate yourself 8-10 feet from the fence on your right side.

If another person drives the horse between you and the fence, you can toss the loop up so the horse runs into it. Keeping the horse along the fence prevents it from dodging away from the rope as you toss it, so the person driving the horse past you must keep it running. The rope can be snubbed around a post to take up the slack when the horse is caught. Because the roped horse may resist violently, it is wise to wear gloves to protect your hands from rope burns.

The halter and lead rope are the main tools of equine restraint, and they should always be used when leading or working on a horse. Check the halter and lead rope for splits or fraying, as a horse can easily break a defective lead rope and/or halter with just a sharp jerk of its head.

Figure 1. Correct positioning for roping a horse.

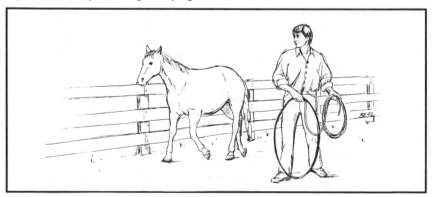

After you have caught the horse and have settled it down, place the neck strap and the buckle end of the halter in your left hand. Standing on the near (left) side, reach your right hand over the horse's neck and take the neck strap from your left hand. Lower your left hand so you do not hit the horse in the nose with the halter as you slide the entire halter back around the horse's neck (Fig 2). Next, gently slide the nose band around the horse's nose and bring the strap over the poll and down the side of the neck; secure the halter by buckling it to the neck strap. Attach the lead rope to the bottom center ring. Check to make sure the halter is settled correctly on the horse's face. There should be no pressure points from rings or rivets, and no straps close to the eyes.

Some horses are "head shy" and throw their heads up or sometimes even rear if a person reaches toward its face. This is usually caused by rough treatment of the horse about the head and neck. To approach this type of horse with the halter, work from the back of the head so the animal does not see the halter approaching. Keep your gestures lower than the muzzle, and move slowly and deliberately. Talk to continually reassure the animal.

If you must approach a horse from the rear, as in a box stall or if the animal is tied, always let the horse know you are approaching. Begin quietly talking before you get close. Remember that a horse's kicking range is 6-8 feet straight back, and

Figure 2A. Reach over the horse's neck and grasp the neck strap.

Figure 2B. Lower the halter so the nose band can be slid up on the nose.

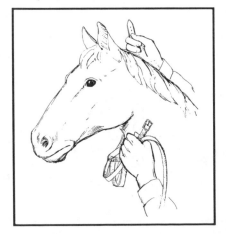

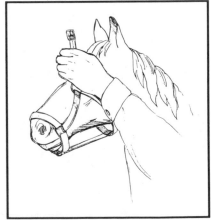

Figure 2C. Hook the neck strap so the halter fits snugly on the horse's face.

Figure 2D. Correct position of the handler's body when holding a horse.

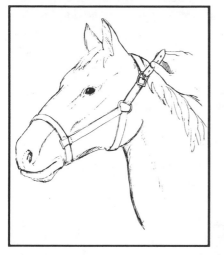
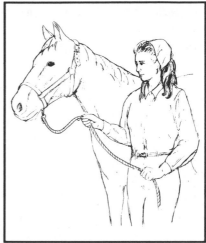

they are usually very accurate. Talk to the horse before and as you approach it, so you do not surprise or startle it. It is safest to pass behind a horse about 10-12 feet or more behind, or to stay in direct physical contact by keeping a hand on the rump when passing around the rear. This does not guarantee that you will not get kicked; however, if you are, the blow will be reduced and further down on your body, where it is less life threatening.

Never get into a very small box stall or small enclosure with a horse. They do not react well to overly constraining conditions, and may panic and trample or kick you in their efforts to get away.

Restraint of Foals

The easiest way to catch a foal is to back the mare into the corner of a large box stall and secure her in place.[2,4] The foal naturally tries to hide behind the mare's flank. When it begins to move, grasp it around the front of the chest with one arm, and quickly around the rump or grasp the tail with the other hand. Once the foal's forward motion is stopped, it typically tries to escape by moving backward.

After you have caught the foal, press it up against the wall or a sturdy partition. If that is not feasible, have another person hold the foal in the same manner on the opposite side. Before capturing the foal, make sure the wall or partition does not have holes through which the foal may put its legs, which could cause injuries.

Do not hold onto the tail too tightly or press it down between the legs, as this sometimes makes the foal sit down. Also, never lift a foal off its feet. This makes them very nervous and they struggle fiercely to regain their feet.

Always talk to and comfort a foal when handling it. Rough handling leads to behavior problems later in life.

Finally, never remove a foal from the sight of its dam. Both dam and foal will fret until they are reunited, and both may injure themselves trying to get back together. Securely tying the dam and keeping the foal within the mare's sight can prevent such problems.

Tying a Horse

The movies would have us believe that a horse will stand quietly in one place until the owner returns, no matter what is going on around it, with only the reins wrapped around a post or dropped to the ground. Unfortunately, this is rarely the case. If a horse is to be left unattended, it should always be tied to a sturdy object with a properly fitting halter and suitable lead rope.

The knot used to tie the lead rope should be a quick-release knot, such as the halter tie (see Chapter 2). The quick-release knot allows the horse to be released quickly if it panics, catches its foot or falls down.

The horse should be allowed about 2-3 feet of lead rope so it can adjust the angle of its neck and shift position as it desires (Fig 3). Allowing more slack than that may cause the horse to tangle its front feet in the rope. Any less slack may frustrate it enough to cause it to try to escape. Do not tie a horse's head too high or too low so it is at an unnatural angle. Rather, tie it so the head is held in a natural position. Always check the

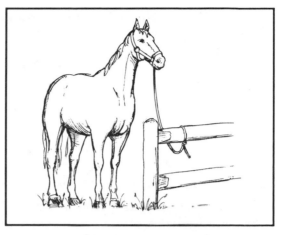

Figure 3. Horse tied to an appropriate height and lead length for safety.

area around a tied horse for possible hazards that could cause serious injuries if the horse were suddenly frightened.

Leading a Horse

Always walk on the near (left) side of the horse, close to the shoulder, and hold the lead rope with your right hand about 1 1/2-2 feet away from the base of the halter. The left hand should hold the loose end of the rope in neat loops, with the entire rope held in front of you. Never wrap the loose end of the lead rope around your hand or have the rope running behind you because if the horse bolts you will be pulled along with it and seriously injured.

After you stop leading a horse, stand as close to the shoulder as possible and face the same direction as the horse (Fig 21). Be careful not to stand too far in front of the horse, as it can rear up and strike with a front foot. Also, do not stand too near or it can accidentally step on the back of your heels as you are walking. Never move under the neck of the horse to get to the other side. This is very dangerous and could result in injury if the horse is suddenly frightened.

Some horses may try to bite you while being led or handled. Punishment should be delivered at the time of the bite by giving a firm rap on the muzzle. You do not usually have to cause pain with such a rap, only convey the impression that you will not tolerate bad behavior. Punishment given too long after the fact is futile.

Restraint of the Head

For almost every veterinary procedure done on a horse, the head must be restrained. The standard equipment for head restraint is the halter and lead rope. They can be used to hold the horse still, direct its attention elsewhere, and secure it to one spot. Therefore, it is very important that this equipment be examined for worn or broken parts before it is used.

Two important rules must be followed when restraining a horse. First, always stand on the same side of the horse as the person who is working on the animal. If the horse tries to escape, it usually will move away from you. If there are people on both sides of it, the animal will pick the smaller of the barriers and move over that. That may result in injury to a person bending or kneeling down.

The second rule is to never stand directly in front of a horse. It can rear up and come down on top of you. It can strike out with its front feet, or can just run you down in an effort to escape. Always stand to the side of the horse and be prepared for a sudden reaction from the horse. Sometimes a halter is not adequate restraint and you must rely on other devices to distract the horse's attention. A twitch or a chain shank may be necessary in such cases.

Twitches

Common types of twitches used on horses are the chain, rope and humane (or clamp) twitches. All have advantages and disadvantages. Often a client's attitude about twitches dictates which one, if any, is used in a particular situation.

The twitch works only for a short time before the muzzle loses feeling, so the greatest effect is when it is first applied. To maximize the twitch's usefulness, tightening and loosening the loop around the muzzle keeps the circulation flowing and keeps the horse's attention on the twitch longer. Be aware that many horses try to get away or resist the twitch when it is first applied; stay with them by moving with their motions.

If they shake you off the first time, it becomes more difficult to place the twitch on again. However, if the horse continues to struggle, try another distraction technique if the horse absolutely resists the twitch.

After the twitch is removed, massage the muzzle to restore circulation. This also lets the horse know that a person can touch its muzzle without hurting it.

The twitch can be applied to the lower lip of a horse as well but should only be used if strong objections are raised by the horse to using the upper lip. Always curl the lip inward to protect the inner surface.

The *chain twitch* is a flat chain loop attached to the end of a stout wooden handle to form a loop. With another person holding onto the horse by means of the halter, hold the twitch handle with your right hand, placing the loop of chain over your left hand and catching one side of the loop between your little finger and ring finger to prevent it from slipping down onto your wrist (Fig 4). Grasp as much of the horse's upper lip with your left hand as possible, pressing the bottom edges together to protect the delicate inner surface, and quickly slide the handle up so the chain loop rests high up around the lip. Tighten the chain around the upper lip by twisting the handle (clockwise if on the left side of the head and counterclockwise if on the right) before letting go of the muzzle (Fig 5).

Periodically tightening and loosening the chain on the muzzle keeps the twitch effective. If steady pressure is constantly applied, the muzzle loses circulation and becomes numb, rendering the twitch ineffective.

An advantage of a chain twitch is that it slips off easily when the chain is loosened. The length of the handle is usually long enough so the restrainer can stand back beside the horse and hang onto the halter as well. The chain can be loosened and tightened or gently wiggled for added distraction. A disadvantage is that some horses learn to wiggle their upper lip to dislodge the twitch.

A *rope twitch* is made from small-diameter cord attached to a stout handle or ring. It is applied to the horse's muzzle in the same manner as a chain twitch.

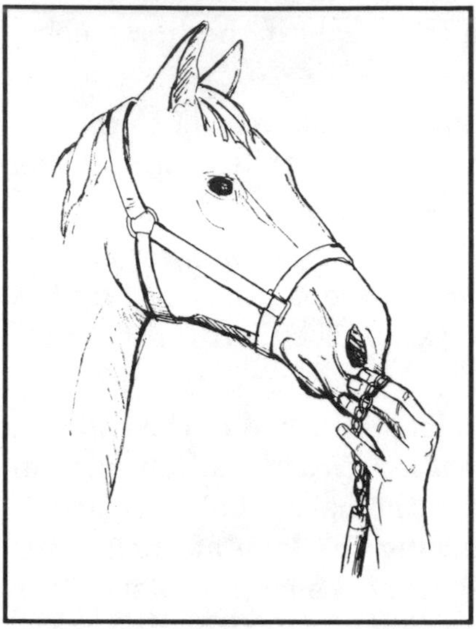

Figure 4. Placing a chain twitch on a horse's upper lip.

Figure 5. Chain twitch in place on a horse's upper lip.

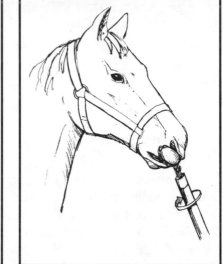

The advantage of a rope twitch is that it is relatively inexpensive and easily made. Also, the loop tends to stay on the horse's muzzle better than a chain. However, this can quickly turn into a disadvantage if the handle is pulled out of the handler's hands by the horse. The free handle can then become a dangerous weapon if the horse throws its head. Another disadvantage of the rope muzzle is that it tends to pinch the horse's muzzle more than the chain, often causing unnecessary pain.

The *humane twitch* is a metal clamp-like device that pinches the upper lip between 2 bars. The twitch usually has a length of cord with a clasp attached to it that can be wrapped around the end of the twitch and then attached to the halter (Fig 6). Regardless of its name, this twitch is not any more humane or inhumane than the chain or rope twitch.

The primary disadvantage of this twitch is that it applies steady pressure that can cause the lip to lose feeling and the twitch to lose its effectiveness. Also, these twitches can be dislodged and become a hazardous flying object because they are attached to the halter.

You can use either hand to grasp the horse's upper lip to apply pressure as a *"manual"* twitch. Do not twist the muzzle, as this causes more pain than is necessary. Simply squeeze or jiggle the muzzle to achieve the desired effect.

Chain Shank

The chain shank is a long leather strap with about 2 ft of flat chain at its end, attached to a snap. It can be used as another distraction device, or on horses that need more restraint than just a halter, such as many stallions. A chain shank can be used in a number of ways.

The first method is the most common. With the halter in place, pass the chain end through the ring on the cheek piece and attach it across the bridge of the nose to the ring on the other side of the head (Fig 7). The chain shank can now be used to keep the horse's attention focused on its nose, to keep the horse under control while leading it, and to prevent it from rearing or trying to bolt.

With the second method, the chain shank is attached in the same places but instead, the chain runs under the jaw. This is really not ideal because this is a very sensitive spot and may cause the horse to throw its head up. The third method is to attach the chain in the same manner but instead of running it over the bridge of the nose, run it between the upper lip and

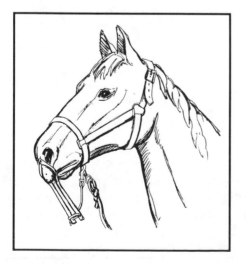

Figure 6. The humane twitch.

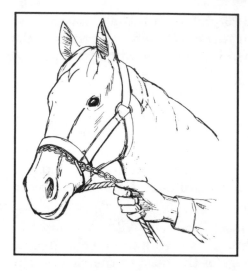

Figure 7. Chain shank across the bridge of the nose.

upper gum (Fig 8). This effectively directs the horse's attention away from other procedures but many horses object strongly to it, and the gums, lips and teeth can be injured.

Figure 8. A. The chain shank is moved between the upper lip and upper front teeth. B. The slack is taken up in the shank. C. Both the shank and lead are grasped in the same hand.

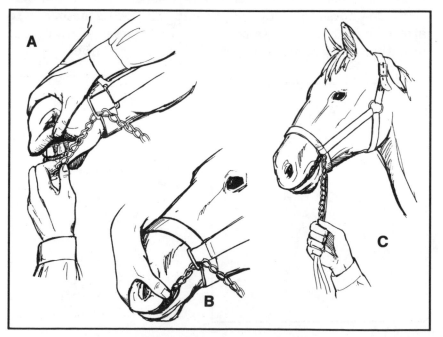

The last method is to run the chain shank through the halter ring on one side and through the mouth like the bit of a bridle, and clip it to the ring on the other side of the halter.

Restraint for Dental Procedures

Restraint for dental procedures involves placing your left hand on the bridge of the nose, with the thumb under the nose band of the halter and the right hand on the nape of the neck (Fig 9).[7,9] This controls the head so the horse is less likely to throw its nose up or suddenly lift the head.

To move the tongue out of the way during a dental procedure, simply hold onto the halter by one of the side straps and gently reach into the mouth at the commissure of the lips with the other hand to grasp the tongue. The 4- to 5-inch interdental space between the incisor teeth and cheek teeth of most horses allows you to reach into the mouth with little danger of being bitten. Gently pull the tongue out of the side of the mouth. The horse may throw its head, so be sure to have a firm hold on the halter.

Figure 9. Technique used to hold the head during dental procedures.

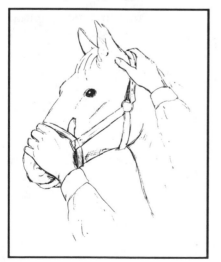

Cross Tying

Cross tying is used to prevent a horse from rearing or from moving the forequarters from side to side.[2,5,8] Remember, however, that a cross-tied horse can still strike with the front feet and move its rear quarters. Cross tying involves placing a second lead rope onto the center ring of the halter and tying one lead to each side of the stanchion or stocks (Fig 10).

Tie the ropes high enough to prevent the horse from rearing and entangling its

Figure 10. Cross tying.

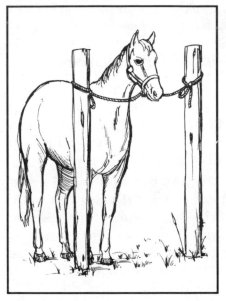

feet in the ropes. The ropes should be wither height or higher, and should only be tied for a short time. If the horse is to be cross tied for a long time, food and water should be elevated so the horse can reach it.

Stocks

Stocks are a narrow enclosure with removable or semi-open sides and a gate at both ends (Fig 11). They can be made of steel pipes or wooden planks, with the top bar or plank no higher than the horse's shoulder. The front of the stocks should have the necessary hooks for cross tying so the horse cannot jump forward or to the side if it tries to escape. A gate is included at both ends because horses do not like narrow, confined areas. The opened front gate gives the appearance of an escape route as the horse is walled into the stocks.

Figure 11. Horse in stocks.

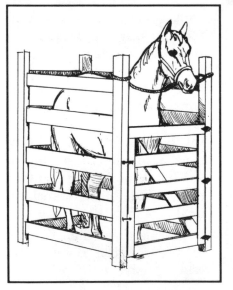

After opening both gates, lead the horse up to the back gate and step to the outside of the stocks. Do not go into the stocks. Pass the rope around the bars as needed to keep the horse moving. Have someone gently close the front and back gates as soon as the horse is properly situated inside. A horse should not be left unattended when placed in stocks.

Hobbles

Breeding hobbles are used to prevent obstinate mares from kicking the stallion while it is trying to mount (Fig 12).[2-4] These hobbles can also be used for rectal or vaginal palpation if stocks are unavailable. Start with a long rope bent in half. Make a bowline on a bight knot (see Chapter 2) and place the loop around the horse's neck, passing both ropes between the front legs. Then pass one rope around each rear leg above the hock. Carry the rope over the standing part, then back around the leg below the hock, from the medial to the lateral side, and pass the end under the rope as it crosses the medial side of the leg. The ends of the rope can be drawn up and tied at the hock or can be taken forward and tied to the halter.

Blindfolds

If a horse is afraid to enter a trailer, stock rack or box stall, or is simply obstinate, a blindfold may help. The blindfolded horse usually calms down and then depends on you to guide it. Work slowly and talk constantly to reassure the blindfolded horse.

Figure 12. Breeding hobbles.

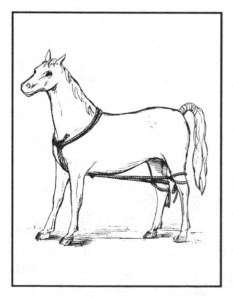

Cradle

A cradle is placed around a horse's neck to prevent chewing or licking at wounds by preventing bending of the neck or turning the head (Fig 13). The cradle must be removed to allow the horse to eat or the food must be raised to head level.

Tail Tie

Much of a horse's weight can be raised or moved by its tail, which is quite strong.

This makes it a handy object to use when you need to move an anesthetized horse. However, the tail can also be a nuisance that must be tied out of the way for certain procedures. Remember to always tie the tail to the animal's own body, as severe injury may result if the tail is tied to an immovable object and the horse suddenly bolts.

To secure a cord or rope to the tail, first find the last coccygeal vertebra of the tail. While supporting the tail in your hand, lay a piece of rope on top of the tail just beyond (caudal to) the last vertebra (Fig 14). The rope should be positioned so the longer end is on the right side of the tail. Fold the rest of the tail up and over the rope. Pass the short end of the rope behind the tail, making a bight as you go. Bring it over the front and pull the bight through the rope that is looped around the tail. The long portion of the rope can now be tied to a front leg or the neck using the bowline knot (see Chapter 2).

Picking Up the Feet

To pick up a front foot, stand parallel to the horse, facing toward the back end. Place one hand on the shoulder and gently but firmly run your other hand down to the fetlock.

Figure 13. Cradle used to prevent self-mutilation.

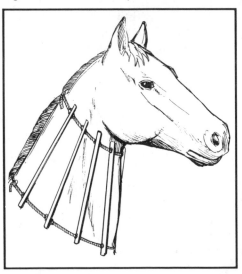

Grasp the fetlock by placing your palm on the underside of the fetlock and wrapping your fingers around the joint. Squeeze and lift the foot at the same time and lean into the horse to make it shift its weight to the other 3 legs. After raising the foot, bring it slightly out to the side, position your body as close in to the horse's body as possible so that your knees are slightly bent, and place the foot

Figure 14. A. First step of the tail tie. B. Position of the ropes for a tail tie. C. The finished tail tie.

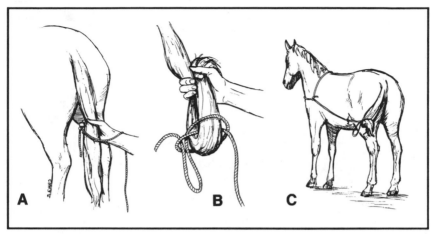

between your legs so that it rests on top of your knees, freeing both of your hands (Fig 15). If the horse jerks its foot, it will usually pull it straight forward, so be ready to stand up if this happens.

The rear feet are approached in the same manner as the front feet. Once you have lifted the foot, extend the leg out to the rear and place it on top of the bent knee closer to the horse (Fig 16). This allows the hands to be free. If the horse moves its foot, it will usually pull back and down off your leg.

Casting

Casting is another term for placing a large animal in lateral recumbency.[4] The old method for casting a large animal, such as a horse, was to use a series of ropes to pull the animal's feet out from underneath it. Use of sedatives and anesthetics makes most manual methods of casting obsolete. The veterinarian is well versed in the different types of injectable drugs that can be used to cast a horse.

Manual Restraint Techniques

If the above restraint methods are not available, manual methods can be used to distract the horse's attention.

Figure 15. Picking up a front foot.   Figure 16. Picking up a back foot.

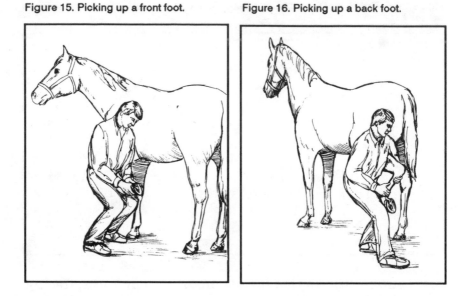

Eye Press

The eye press involves gently placing a finger on the upper eyelid and pressing down. This may be difficult and undesirable if the horse is head shy. Never reach directly toward the eye because this could make the horse throw its head. Work your way up to the eye by slowly moving your hand up the side of the face.

Shoulder Roll

To apply a shoulder roll, grasp a large fold of skin with both hands just over the shoulder. Wiggling and moving it from side to side or up and down provides excellent distraction.

Petting

"Caveman pets" or somewhat heavy swats sometimes provide all the distraction necessary for minor procedures. It is also helpful to talk to the animal in a firm but soothing voice while using all these techniques.

Foot Elevation

The last technique is useful if the horse does not want to stand still when a radiograph is being made or a bandage is being applied or removed. Position the horse where you want it and then pick up or tie up the opposite foot from the one being radiographed or bandaged. A horse rarely wants to move with only 3 feet on the ground.

Grasping the Ear

Some people advocate grasping the base of the ear with the heel of your hand touching the head and squeezing the ear to divert the horse's attention. If you use this technique, be sure that you do not apply excessive pressure to the ear, as damage to the cartilage can cause the ear to permanently flop over. Another disadvantage to this technique is that it may make the horse afraid to have its ears touched, which can cause the owner of a show animal a lot of frustration when the hair on the ears must be trimmed. This technique should only be used with the owner's permission.

References

1. Blanchard S: Here's how to read your horse's body language. *Pet Health News* May:25, 1984.

2. Fowler ME: *Restraint and Handling of Wild and Domestic Animals.* Iowa State Univ Press, Ames, 1978. pp 93-112.

3. Leahy JR and Barrow P: *Restraint of Animals.* Cornell Campus Store, Ithaca, NY, 1953. pp 38-85.

4. Neil DH and Kese ML, in McCurnin DM: *Clinical Textbook for Veterinary Technicians.* Saunders, Philadelphia, 1985. pp 8-16.

5. Nelson B: Restraining horses. *Western Horseman* October:89-94, 1980.

6. Strickland C: How to tie your horse safely and securely. *Horse Illustrated* May:39-43, 1988.

7. Vail C: Tips on Equine dentistry. *Norden News* Summer:15-17, 1980.

8. Vanderhurst SR, in Catcott EJ: *Animal Health Technology.* American Veterinary Publications, Goleta, CA, 1977. pp 355-361.

9. Vaughan JT and Allen R: Restraint of horses: Part I - Head restraint. *Modern Veterinary Practice* 68:373-383, 1987.

6

Restraint of Cattle

The type of restraint used on cattle depends on the animal's breed, age and sex.[1,3,4] Is it a calf, steer, beef cow, dairy cow or bull? The handling necessary for different cattle is also influenced by their previous exposure to people.

Dairy cows are accustomed to being touched and having people around them. In contrast, beef cattle may only see people twice a year, and then they may be subjected to some painful procedures. All bulls, both beef and dairy, are very unpredictable and should always be handled very cautiously. Dairy bulls are especially unpredictable and can kill a careless handler.

Signs of aggression in bulls include pawing the ground with the front feet, and lowering and shaking the head. Nervous cows keep their head and tail up, and have a somewhat wild look in their eyes.

Herding Cattle

Cattle are often treated as a herd. If driven in the proper manner, they are easily moved from one place to another.[2] It is best to keep them as calm as possible so that they do not run. Once they are "spooked" it is difficult to settle them down enough so you can direct their movements or accomplish the intended procedures. Urging by voice and judicious use of a whip or prod only on the rump and back of the legs are the best ways to keep a herd moving and under control.

When the herd is near the barn or pen into which they must go, do not push them too hard. Rather, allow them to look inside and inspect the area. If you do not allow them to look the place over, usually they scatter in every direction and will not enter the enclosure.

It is difficult to separate a cow and her calf away from the herd because they instinctively try to remain with the herd for protection. Cutting a small group of cows and calves from the herd, including the one you want, is much easier.

Restraint in Chutes

A chute is usually used to restrain beef cattle and bulls. Most dairy cows are treated in a stanchion. The chute is usually at the end of an alleyway that allows only one animal access to the chute. To the animal, the chute appears as a continuation of the alley. When the animal reaches the neck squeeze area, the neck is caught by gates closed by the handler or contact with the animal's shoulders (Fig 1).

A rear gate is often closed to prevent other animals from entering the chute and to prevent the animal from backing out

Figure 1. Cow in one type of chute. Notice the squeeze panel, which restricts lateral movement. Not shown is a gate that swings out to allow one to get close to the cow after catching the head.

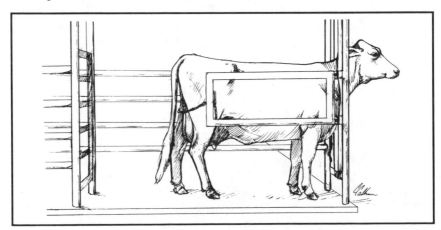

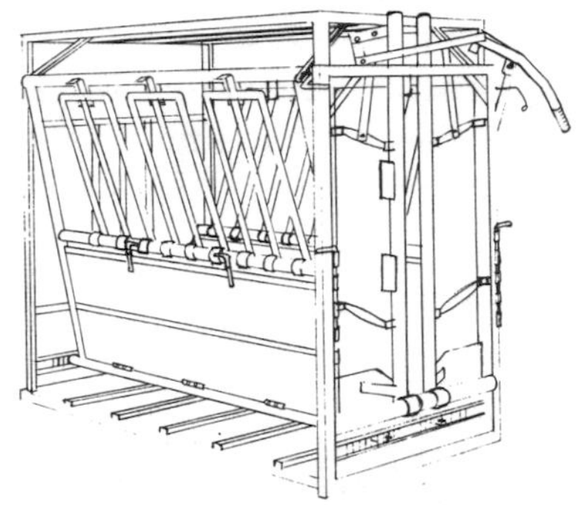

Figure 2. Squeeze chute with bars that can be lowered to give injections and a lower panel that can fold down to allow work on the feet.

of the chute. For further restraint, the walls on some types of chutes squeeze in or gates are used to push the animal to one side of the chute. Squeezing should be the last step in the capture process.

Some chutes have side panels that fold down to allow work on the feet, or side bars that can be dropped to examine the body or give vaccinations (Fig 2). The neck squeeze allows the head and eyes to be examined or oral medications to be administered. The tail gate protects the veterinarian during rectal or vaginal examination. If the chute does not have a tail gate, place a plank, pipe or stack of bales behind the rear legs of the animal to prevent it from kicking the veterinarian.

To release an animal from the chute, the operation is reversed. The body squeeze is released, the neck squeeze is opened wide and the animal is chased out of the chute. Always ready the chute for the next animal before opening the rear gate. This prevents an anxious animal from charging through the chute before you are ready to catch it.

Time can be saved and injuries avoided if you familiarize yourself with operation of the chute before using it.

Restraint of the Head

Most head restraint can be applied after the animal is caught in a chute.[1-4] Restraining the animal in a chute makes it easier for the handler to catch the head and avoid injury. This is not to say that you cannot be injured once the animal is in a chute. Cattle in a chute can still swing their head in a fairly high and wide arc. Cattle with horns can do considerable damage. For this reason, always approach the animal from the side because approaching directly from the front may be construed as a challenge, and the animal may try to butt you.

Rope Halter

A rope halter is the best tool for restraining the head of a cow. A properly placed halter will not injure the animal if it must be tied for a long period, and the halter is strong enough to restrain the head.

To apply the halter, locate the noseband, which is the portion of the halter that tightens when you pull on the loose end. This should go around the nose (muzzle). The head stall is the longer loop that goes around the back of the animal's head.

Stand on the left side of the animal and place the nose band around the muzzle, with the portion that tightens under the chin and the loose end coming out of the left side. Place the head stall behind the ears. Do not leave the head stall in front of the ears, as the halter could slip off. Check the halter for a proper fit (Fig 3). No part of the halter should be close to or over the eyes. If it is, pull on the nose band to pull it forward, being careful not to pull it farther forward than the nasal bones because the rope could block off the air passages. The animal's head may now be manipulated for examination of the eyes, ears or mouth, or for jugular venipuncture.

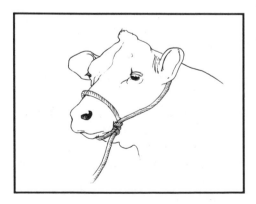

Figure 3. Rope halter properly placed on a steer.

Mouth Speculum

To administer oral medication, a mouth speculum can be used to hold the mouth open so the animal does not bite down on the stomach tube or balling gun. To place the speculum, first apply a halter, then stand to the side of the head. Reach around the mandible and grasp it with your hand, resting the head on your thigh. With your other hand, reach into the animal's mouth at the commissure of the lips, gently pry open the mouth, and quickly slide in the speculum (Fig 4).

Nose Lead

The nose lead restrains cattle by applying pressure to the nasal septum. The nose lead is shaped like a pair of tongs, with a large ball at the end of each arm that fits up against the nasal septum. It is important to frequently check the balls for rough edges, as they can tear the nasal mucosa. Also, if the balls press against each other when the instrument is applied, circulation to the nasal septum is interrupted and the lead becomes ineffective.

To place the nose lead, first hold the lead out for the animal to sniff. When the animal raises its head to sniff, slip one ball of the lead into one nostril and quickly move the other ball

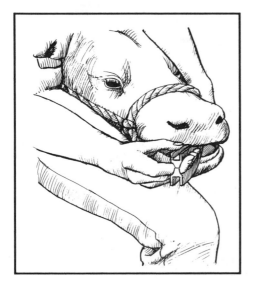

Figure 4. Inserting a speculum into a cow's mouth.

into the other nostril, closing the 2 pieces together. Most leads have a chain or rope attached so the animal's head can be tied up and to the side for examination or jugular venipuncture. A halter tie, snubbing hitch or some other quick-release knot is used so the nose lead can quickly be released if the animal falls down (Fig 5).

Another way to place the nose lead is to stand to the side of the animal's head. Reach around the muzzle with your hand and pull the head up by holding onto the mandible. Slip the nose lead on and tie it as described.

Animals that have been repeatedly restrained by a nose lead become increasingly head shy. Therefore, it is better to routinely use the halter because of its less traumatic nature, and only use a nose lead when necessary.

Nose Ring

Most dairy bulls have permanent nose rings placed through their nasal septum. Two methods are used to handle bulls. The first involves use of a bull staff, which is a long rod with a hook on the end. The rod is attached to the nose ring and, along with the halter, is used to lead the bull.

The second method is to attach 2 lead ropes to the nose ring, with one person on either end and one handler in control of the halter (Fig 6). This cross-tying effect is usually considered the safest method of handling a bull.

The nose ring can help control a dairy bull but should never be considered foolproof.

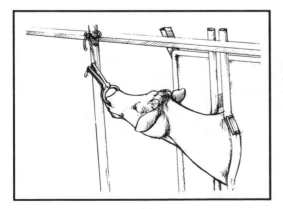

Figure 5. Cow in a squeeze chute, with a nose lead tied by a halter tie.

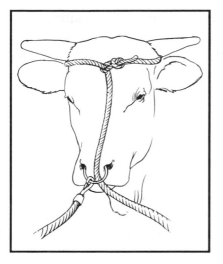

Figure 6. Cross-tying a bull with a nose ring.

Restraint Using the Tail

The tail of cattle is not nearly as strong as that of horses. It cannot support the animal's weight, and breaks easily if handled roughly. Despite these limitations, "jacking" the tail is useful to distract cattle from painful procedures done elsewhere on the body.[2-4]

To jack the tail, place the animal in a chute or stanchion and grasp the tail as close to its base as possible. Use both hands to gently ease the tail vertically (Fig 7). Such procedures as rectal or vaginal examination, coccygeal venipuncture or udder examination can be performed with the tail in this position.

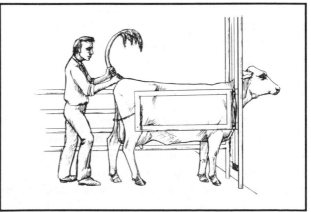

Figure 7. Tail jacking a cow in a squeeze chute.

It is very important to keep the tail along the midline and not deflected to one side. If it is deflected to one side, this makes the animal move forward, or you may fracture a vertebra in the tail. When the procedure is done, the tail should be lowered carefully. Do not simply drop it.

Tail Tying

Some dairy cows swing their tail into your face or keep it in the way as you work near their hindquarters. Tail tying, as described for horses (see Chapter 5), works equally well for cattle. Remember to always tie the tail to the animal's own body and not to an immovable object. Tying the tail to a fixed object can result in a fracture or avulsion of the switch at the end of the tail if the animal bolts.

Some beef cattle accumulate plant fibers or other debris in the switch at the end of the tail. To remove cockleburs and other plant fibers, soak the tail in mineral oil and comb the switch out. Try not to pull too much hair out, as this is the animal's only means of swatting flies. The hair eventually grows back if any is pulled out.

Restraint of the Legs

In addition to butting, another defensive mechanism of cattle is kicking. Most cattle do not usually kick straight backward like a horse. Rather, they usually kick in a forward motion that then arcs backward. The safest place to stand is next to the shoulder, but be aware that cattle can kick past their shoulder with their rear legs, though the force is diminished. Restraining the feet of cattle for trimming or treatment of the hooves frequently requires sedation or general anesthesia, and use of a hydraulic tilt table.

Hobbles

Various types of hobbles are available to prevent an animal from kicking. Milking or chain hobbles have 2 metal bands that are bent to fit around the leg just proximal to (above) the hock (Fig 8). To apply them, stand on the cow's right side, facing toward the rear. Squat down and apply the left hobble

Figure 8. Milking hobbles.   Figure 9. Rope hobbles.

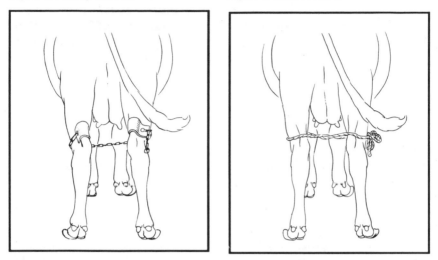

first, then the right. Be ready to move out of the way if the cow decides to kick before the hobbles are in place. The chain should pass around the front of the legs and should be adjusted so the animal can maintain its balance.

A small-diameter rope may also be used as a hobble. Stand on the animal's right side and place the rope around the left rear leg just proximal to (above) the hock. Position the rope so that both end segments are the same length. Cross the rope once between the legs and bring the ends around the right leg. Tie the ends in a bow for quick release (Fig 9).

Flank Rope

Another method of preventing kicking is to tie a small-diameter rope around the animal's flank. Be careful when positioning and tightening the rope on dairy cows and bulls, because the rope passes over the udder and prepuce, respectively, and could damage them if applied too tightly.

Restraint of Calves

Beef and dairy calves can be handled in much the same manner. Dairy heifer calves should not be handled roughly, as this may result in a bad-tempered adult cow.

Always be very careful when working with a calf in the presence of its dam. Cows are very protective and may charge you. A cow can kill a person with a single blow of her head to the chest. If the cow is with her calf, it is a simple matter of moving the cow in the desired direction. The calf will follow. To move the calf to another pen or enclosure without the cow, wrap one arm around the front of the calf's chest. With the other hand, control the back end by holding the calf's tail or the rear quarters (Fig 10). A larger calf can be led by using a rope halter, but this often results in a tug of war. It is easier to treat larger calves like adults and simply herd them to the desired area.

Flanking

Flanking, or placing a calf in lateral recumbency, is easy if you position yourself properly. Place the calf's body so its left side is parallel to your legs. Position your right knee into the calf's flank and reach around the calf's body to grasp the opposite flank with the right hand. With the left hand, grasp the loose skin just behind the shoulder. Push into the calf with your knee and lift up with both hands at the same time, letting the calf slide down your legs to break the fall. Follow the calf down and place one knee on the neck.

Quickly gather up the back legs and the top front leg, and tie them together (Fig 11). The tie commonly used is a loop placed around all 3 legs. Wrap the cord around the legs twice

Figure 10. Restraint of a calf.

Figure 11. Tying a calf's legs together after it has been flanked.

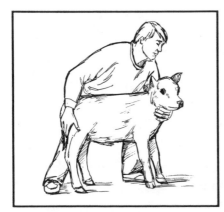

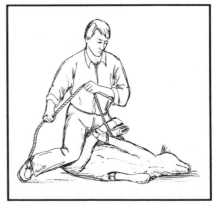

and secure with a half hitch and then another half hitch that includes a bight for easy removal.

References

1. Aanes WA: Restraint of cattle: Head restraint. *Modern Veterinary Practice* 68:498-501, 1987.

2. Fowler ME: *Restraint and Handling of Wild and Domestic Animals.* Iowa State Univ Press, Ames, 1978. pp 113-130.

3. Leahy JR and Barrow P: *Restraint of Animals.* Cornell Campus Store, Ithaca, NY, 1953. pp 86-125.

4. Neil DH and Kese ML, in McCurnin DM: *Clinical Textbook for Veterinary Technicians.* Saunders, Philadelphia, 1985. pp 16-18.

5. Vanderhurst SR and Hunter RL, in Catcott EJ: *Animal Health Technology.* American Veterinary Publications, Goleta, CA, 1977. pp 347-348.

7

Restraint of Pigs

Pigs are generally intelligent, stubborn, contrary, vocal and sometimes downright vicious animals.[1-3] These traits make them one of the most difficult animals to restrain without injury to yourself or to the pig. Though pigs seem like hardy animals, they have some physical disadvantages. Poor eyesight makes them easily frightened. An insulating layer of fat makes them susceptible to hyperthermia if treated too roughly for long periods. Small-boned legs can break easily if grasped or tied in the wrong manner. For this reason, you must move slowly and deliberately when handling pigs. Talk to reassure the animals and handle them as gently as possible.

Their primary means of defense is their sharp teeth, which even in newborn pigs can cause much damage. Their snout and shoulder and neck muscles are very strong allowing them to lift heavy panels of fencing.

With their streamlined bodies they can also squeeze through small openings. This can be quite dangerous if the pig is angry, and lifts fence panels and squeezes through openings to chase you. Pigs' streamlined bodies also make them difficult to hold with bare hands, so ropes or other restraint tools must be used. Working quickly, quietly and efficiently minimizes the possibility of injury to you and the pig.

Moving and Capturing Pigs

It is nearly impossible to capture one pig out of a herd because they cannot be herded like cows or sheep.[1-4] Other pigs may come to the aid of a squealing herdmate and they may become aggressive without much warning.

The safest method for capturing a single pig from a herd is to move all of the pigs into a small pen using barriers or hurdles. Hurdles are flat pieces of plywood, plastic or metal large enough to cover your legs (Fig 1). Some are equipped with handles or holes cut into them so you can easily carry them in front of you. Hurdles can be used to crowd the pigs into a pen or to set up temporary fences while the pigs are moved from place to place. They are also used to isolate a particular pig after the herd has been moved into a smaller pen.

If a pig tries to go under the hurdle, pull the top of the hurdle toward you. You can also slap the pig on the snout to stop its forward momentum, but be careful not to slap it too hard. This can have the opposite effect, angering the animal so it becomes aggressive. For this reason, before working with a pig or group of pigs, plan possible escape routes you can use if a pig becomes aggressive.

Pigs can be directed with a flat stick or cane (Fig 2). Gently tapping the pig on the shoulder or side of the face turns the animal in the desired direction. Do not use the cane to inflict

Figure 1. Hurdle used to direct a pig's movement.

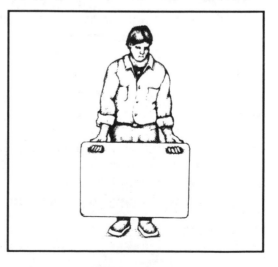

Figure 2. Using a cane to direct a pig's movement.

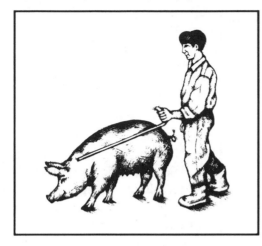

pain, as you can enrage the pig and it may come after you. You may also damage its body with severe blows.

Pigs can also be maneuvered with a rope harness. Make a loop that can be passed over the pig's head and tightened in front of the shoulders. Then make a half hitch in the standing part of the rope. Hold the loop down in front of the pig so it can walk through the loop. When the front legs have passed through the loop, pull the rope tight (Fig 3). By applying different pressures to the rope you can maneuver the pig where you want it.

Carrying or Lifting Pigs

Pigs weighing under 50 lb can be restrained for vaccination, castration or administration of medication by lifting them by the rear or front feet. To restrain for castration or axillary and inguinal vaccination, capture the pig by a rear leg proximal to (above) the hock. Grasp a rear leg in each hand and lift the body, placing the head between your legs (Fig 4). Let the front legs touch the ground to support some of the animal's weight, and to help calm it. If the vaccination is to

Figure 3. Using a rope harness to control the actions of a pig.

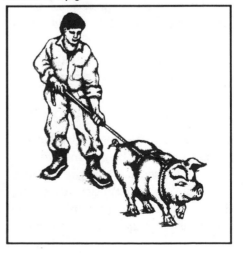

Figure 4. Restraint for castration or vaccination of a pig weighing under 50 lb.

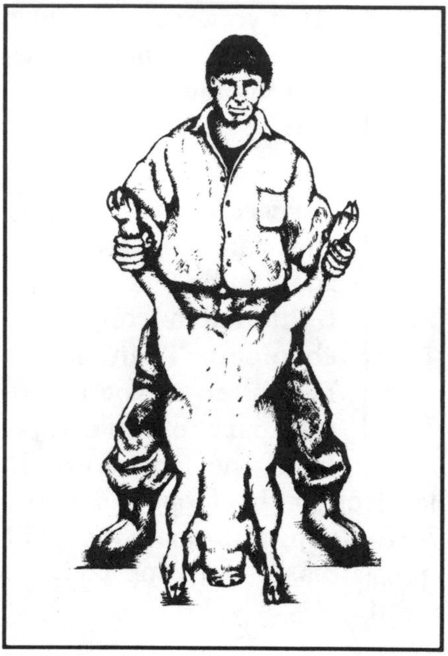

be given behind the ear or on the shoulder, or if medication is to be given orally, catch the pig in the same manner but elevate the front legs off the ground, letting the animal's shoulders and back rest against your legs for support.

Newborn pigs can be quickly lifted by the tail. With older piglets up to 4 lb, include a rear leg in your grasp to prevent tail injury. Piglets over 4 lb can be grasped by a rear leg. Then quickly place one hand under the chest and the other over the shoulders (Fig 5). Holding them firmly but gently in this manner usually calms them and stops their squealing.

Be prepared to move quickly if the piglets squeal and the sow is near. A sow with a litter should be assumed to be aggressive. She may try to climb over the farrowing crate or go under it to come to the defense of her piglets. For this reason, it is best to move the piglets to another room to work on them, as their squealing can cause the sow to become aggressive.

Restraint of the Head

Most of the restraint procedures on adult pigs involve the head.[1-4] Because the pig is such a predictably stubborn creature, its stubbornness can be used to your advantage. Pigs naturally

Figure 5. Proper way to hold a piglet.

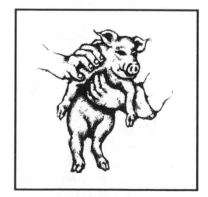

move in a direction opposite to the one in which they are steered. By pulling in the opposite direction, we can usually make them move in the desired direction.

Bucket

To move an individual pig to a particular spot, place a bucket over the head. The pig naturally backs away from the bucket. By holding onto the tail and steering the pig, you can move the animal as needed (Fig 6).

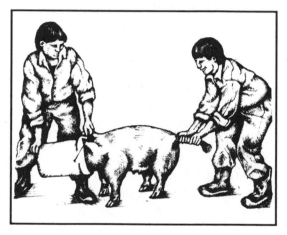

Figure 6. Placing a bucket over the pig's head allows you to direct its backward movement by guiding with the tail.

Snubbing Rope

A snubbing rope works well to hold a pig in one spot or to tie a pig to a fence. Make a loop in a short length of rope. Stand close behind the pig and dangle the loop in front of the animal's face. When the pig begins to mouth the rope, quickly pull the rope into the mouth as close to the commissure of the lips as possible, and tighten the loop across the top of the pig's snout (Fig 7). The rope must be looped

Figure 7. Snubbing rope used to control a pig.

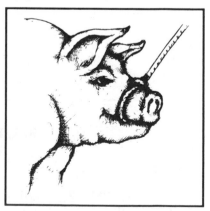

behind the tusks, which may be difficult on a boar with large tusks. A hog snare works better on these animals (see below).

If the pig will not mouth the rope, the loop can be forced into the pig's mouth by grasping both sides of the loop and sawing the rope back and forth. Once the rope is in the mouth, apply steady pressure and move to the front of the pig. The animal naturally pulls against this forward pressure, and the rope may now be tied to a fence. *Do not leave the animal unattended*, as it may chew through the rope. Do not leave the rope on for more than 15-20 minutes because of its tourniquet-like effect on the snout.

If a pig violently resists a single rope, another snubbing rope can be placed into the pig's mouth and the pig can be cross tied.

Hog Snare

A hog snare is the restraint tool of choice when restraining a large pig. The principle is the same as for the snubbing rope. The snare is usually a metal pipe with a cable loop on one end. The free end of the cable runs through the hollow pipe so the size of the loop can be controlled (Fig 8). The loop is dangled in front of the pig. When the pig has the loop in its mouth behind the tusks, the loop is tightened. Be careful not to apply excessive pressure to the pig's snout, as the cable may damage it.

Figure 8. Hog snare.

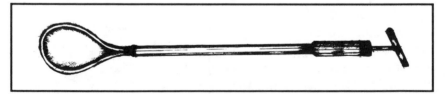

Casting Pigs

Hobbles

There are various ways to cast pigs. All involve initially gaining control of the pig's head with a snubbing rope or

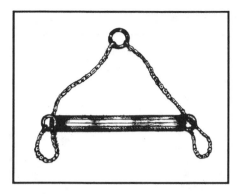

Figure 9. Hog hobbles, used in lateral recumbency.

snare. One method involves use of hobbles specifically designed for pigs (Fig 9). After gaining control of the head, place the hobbles on the back legs, attach a rope to the hobble and pull the rear legs out from under the pig. Gently twist so the pig is thrown off balance.

Another method involves using the standing part of the snubbing rope. After securing the snubbing rope to the pig's snout, use a half hitch to secure one of the rear legs. Now pull up on the rope to draw the pig's foot and nose together, knocking the animal off its feet (Fig 10).

The last method is to attach a rope to a front and rear leg on one side of the pig. Pass both ropes under the abdomen and

Figure 10. Placing a pig in lateral recumbency using a snubbing rope.

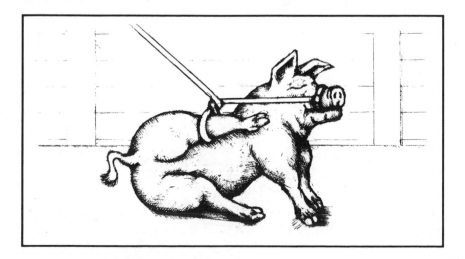

Figure 11. First step in placing a pig in lateral recumbency.

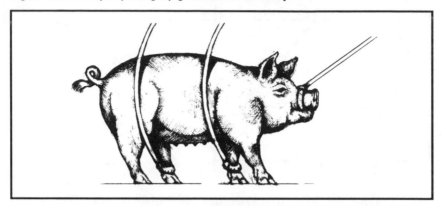

up the opposite side of the pig and then over the back, toward you. Pulling up on the ropes pulls the feet out from under the pig, toppling it over on its side (Fig 11). The ropes can then be used to tie the legs together (Fig 12).

Trough

A restraint tool that can be used to keep smaller pigs on their backs is a V-shaped trough. Place the pig in the trough on its back. Tie a small-diameter rope around the pig's rear foot, run the rope beneath the trough to the other side and attach it to the other foot. Repeat the procedure with the front feet. This keeps the pig in place so the trough can be tilted in any direction (Fig 13).

Figure 12. Last step in placing a pig in lateral recumbency.

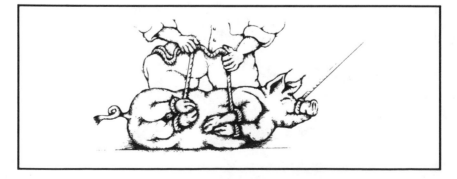

Figure 13. Small pig restrained in a trough.

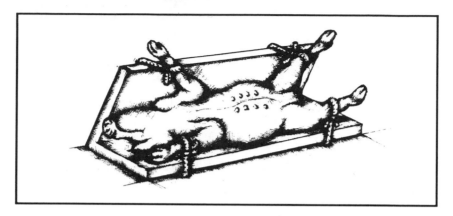

References

1. Fowler ME: *Restraint and Handling of Wild and Domestic Animals.* Iowa State Univ Press, Ames, 1978. pp 139-147.

2. Kocab JM: Restraint of pigs. *New Methods* February:12-13, 1983.

3. Leahy JR and Barrow P: *Restraint of Animals.* Cornell Campus Store, Ithaca, NY, 1953. pp 126-163.

4. Neil DH and Kese ML, in McCurnin DM: *Clinical Textbook for Veterinary Technicians.* Saunders, Philadelphia, 1985. pp 19-20.

8

Restraint of Sheep

Sheep are very easy creatures to restrain if you consider their intense instinct to remain with the flock. This is their main means of defense. By moving as a flock, each member has a better chance of escaping danger. If one sheep requires treatment, the flock is stressed less if the entire flock is allowed to move into a small pen together and the individual needing treatment is then removed.

Sheep show that they are disturbed by stamping their front feet or butting with their head. Rams are especially fond of butting and do so with little provocation, particularly during breeding season.

Always work gently, calmly and with assurance around sheep. Sheep can be severely injured by improper restraint. They have very fragile bones that can be easily broken by a careless handler. Therefore, be aware of this when you grasp a body part.

Sheep with a full coat of wool can become hyperthermic if they are chased. Also, if the wool is pulled out in a struggle, the fleece is reduced in value. Even if the fleece is not pulled out but just pulled on, a subcutaneous bruise can reduce the carcass value.

Figure 1. Capturing and holding a sheep.

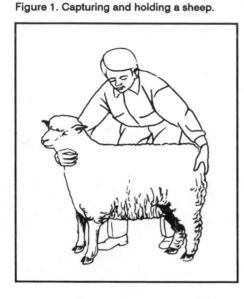

Capturing Sheep

The easiest way to separate an individual from the flock is to drive the flock into a small pen or enclosure.[1-4] Approach the individual slowly. When you are close, swing your arm around the neck and front quarters, and quickly wrap your other arm around the rear quarters, grasping the dock (tail) (Fig 1). This method of restraint allows you to steer the animal into another pen or move it to a treatment area.

A shepherd's crook can also be used to capture a sheep by hooking a back leg in the area of the hock (Fig 2). Hook and immobilize the animal quickly so it does not have an opportunity to fight the crook and possibly break a leg. Do not use the crook around the neck or more distally on the leg, as it can cause severe damage.

Halters can be used on sheep; however, they have a short nose and you must be careful that the nose band does not slip down and occlude the nostrils.

Figure 2. Use of a shepherd's crook to capture a sheep.

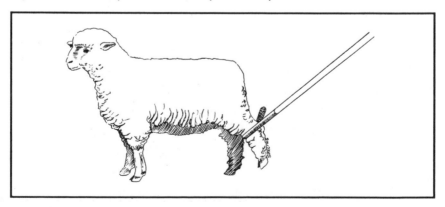

Restraint for Examination

If the dorsal aspect of the body is to be examined, hooves trimmed, wool sheered or a subcutaneous vaccination given, the easiest method of restraint is to set the animal up on its rump. Most sheep do not seem to object strongly to this. It is relatively easy to flip a sheep onto its rump. One of the easiest ways is to stand on the left side of the animal with its body parallel to your legs (Fig 3).

Place your left knee against the shoulder. With your right hand, grasp the flank on the right side of the sheep. Hold the jaw with your left hand. Move the sheep's head to the right toward its shoulder and, at the same time, step back with your right leg and lift up the flank. This throws the sheep off balance. With a quick twist you can set it up on its rump (Fig 4). Then move behind the sheep so your legs can brace the sheep's back. Tilting the animal back so it is sitting at about a 60-degree angle keeps it from struggling to right itself. Be careful of the front legs, as some sheep flail them about and could injure your face.

Restraint for Medication

Oral medication for sheep typically is in the form of individual boluses or a drenching solution. The easiest method of delivering this type of medication is to run a few head of sheep into a squeeze pen or small box stall so there is little or no room for movement. Then wade in among them. Grasp the jaw to elevate the head so it is nearly perpendicular to the ground.

Figure 3. Correct placement of the hands in preparation for setting a sheep on its rump.

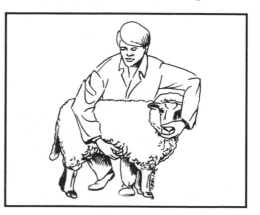

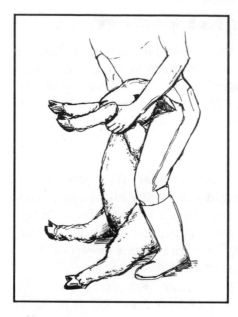

Figure 4. Setting a sheep on its rump.

After the medication is given, lower the head somewhat to allow the animal to swallow. A marking crayon should be used to mark each sheep after it has been medicated. This prevents double dosing. To medicate a single sheep in a pen, back the animal into a corner. If you are tall enough, straddle it and give the medication. If the sheep is too tall, back it into a corner, reach around the opposite side of the neck and hold the head so that you can give the medication (Fig 5).

Figure 5. Restraint for drenching, balling or jugular venipuncture.

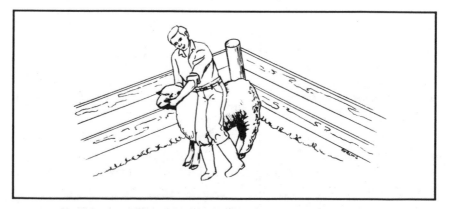

Restraint for Jugular Venipuncture

Sheep stocks greatly facilitate restraint for jugular venipuncture (Fig 6). The head is restrained and lateral movements are restricted quite well with the animal in stocks.
However, many farms do not have stocks, and it is necessary
to manually restrain the sheep for venipuncture.

Start by capturing the sheep in the method described for
medicating. Maneuver the sheep around so its rear quarters
are in a corner and one side is against the wall. Then straddle
the animal and grasp the mandible, one side in each hand.
Gently elevate the sheep's head. If the sheep is too tall to
straddle, push the sheep sideways against the wall and stand
on the opposite side. Keep the sheep against the wall with
your legs and hold the head up as described (Fig 5).

Jugular venipuncture is also possible with the sheep set up
on its rump. Tuck the head below your elbow to restrain it.

Figure 6. Sheep restrained in stocks for jugular venipuncture.

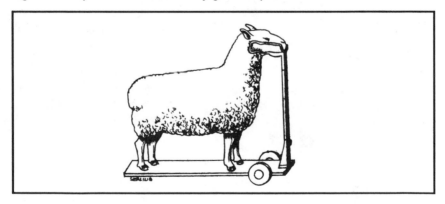

Restraint of Lambs

Newborn lambs are easily carried by placing your hand between their front legs, with the sternum resting on your forearm (Fig 7). Large lambs are handled as adults.

Restraint for castration and tail docking is relatively easy.
The lambs should be placed in a small pen so you do not have
to chase them around to capture them. After you have captured one, grasp the front leg and rear leg on the same side in

Figure 7. Carrying newborn and small lambs.

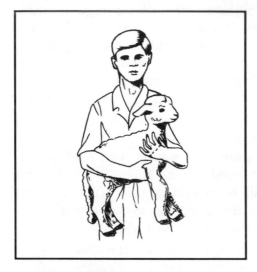

Figure 8. Restraint of a lamb for castration and tail docking.

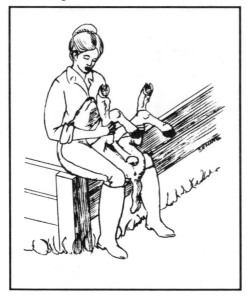

each hand, right hand grasping right side, left hand grasping left side, and flip the animal onto its back (Fig 8). The lamb's back should rest against your chest or lap if you are sitting down. Tilt the lamb back to expose the tail and scrotum.

References

1. Faler K and Faler K: Restraint of sheep. *Modern Veterinary Practice* 68:562-563, 1987.

2. Fowler ME: *Restraint and Handling of Wild and Domestic Animals.* Iowa State Univ Press, Ames, 1978.

3. Leahy JR and Barrow P: *Restraint of Animals.* Cornell Book Store, Ithaca, NY, 1953.

4. Neil DH and Kese ML, in McCurnin DM: *Clinical Textbook for Veterinary Technicians.* Saunders, Philadelphia, 1985. pp 18-19.

9

Restraint of Goats

Goats do not tolerate rough treatment and will struggle violently if improperly handled. For this reason, the minimum amount of restraint necessary to complete the medical procedure should be used.

Contrary to popular belief, goats cannot be treated like sheep. They do not have the same strong instincts to remain with a group as do sheep, and are more likely to scatter if you try to herd them.[1-4] It is better to identify the lead goat, usually a nanny, and lead her into the barn or pen; the rest of the goats will likely follow.

Goats are usually docile and easily handled. However, you must be friendly or they will become agitated and try to butt you. Signs of impending aggression include holding the tail close to the back with the hair raised along the spine, sneezing, snorting and stamping. If these signals are ignored, the goat may rear up on its hind legs and butt you.

Restraint for Examination

To capture a goat and have it remain still, grasp a front leg and lift it (Fig 1). Most goats stand peacefully when restrained in this way, allowing most types of procedures to be done. This technique works well with both large and small goats. The rear leg can be used for capturing goats, but it is not a good re-

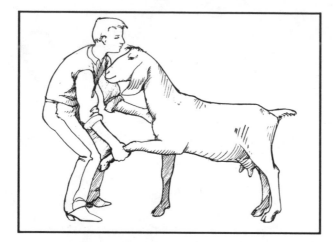

Figure 1. Restraint capture to prevent a goat from moving.

straint technique, as the goat usually kicks out and struggles. Sometimes, however, the hind leg is the only way to capture a goat. Once the animal is caught, another restraint technique should then be used.

Walls or fences can be used to help restrain a goat for short medical procedures. Push the goat's body against the fence or wall with your legs and hips, leaving your hands free for the procedure. Placing the goat's hindquarters toward a corner is another good technique. Placing one arm around the goat's neck keeps it still. This works well for injections and for determining the animal's temperature, pulse and respiratory rate.

Unlike sheep, goats resent being set up on their rump. They lash out with the front legs and are usually agile enough to squirm out of the hold. A better method is to lay the goat on its side or flank it.

There are 2 methods for flanking a goat. The first positions the goat's body parallel to your legs. Grasp the nose with one hand and the inside (near) rear leg with the other. Bring the leg forward and the nose back to meet the leg (Fig 2). This throws the goat off balance, causing it to fall to the ground.

The second method also positions the goat's body parallel to your legs. Reach over the goat's back and down beneath its abdomen to grasp the near legs. Lift the legs and gently flop the goat down onto the ground. Once the goat is down, firmly hold

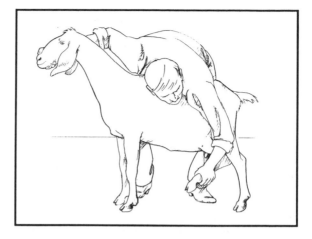

Figure 2. Initial step in flanking a goat.

all 4 legs and gently press your knee on the neck to keep the animal recumbent.

Restraint of the Head

Head restraint is necessary for eye examinations, giving oral medication or jugular venipuncture.[2-4] The technique used depends on your preference or the circumstances. Head restraint techniques work best if the goat is backed into a corner and pushed sideways against the wall. This keeps the animal from backing up or moving to the side.

The first technique involves grasping the beard with one hand and encircling the neck with the other arm to stabilize the head (Fig 3). Most goats do not object to this technique, though there is a disadvantage to it. During mating season, male goats urinate on their beards to attract females. This strong odor tends to permeate your clothing and skin.

In the second method, the horns are used to capture and lead the goat for short distances. However, you should switch to a different hold as soon as possible because goats resent having their horns handled and may butt or lash out with their feet.

The head can also be controlled by placing one hand on either side of the cheeks, wrapping your fingers around the mandible and holding firmly (Fig 4). This stabilizes the head for jugular venipuncture and eye examination.

Figure 3. Beard and neck hold for general examination.

Figure 4. Cheek hold for general examination and jugular venipuncture.

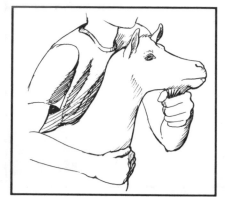
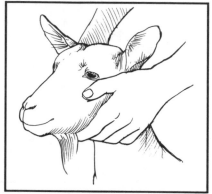

Collars

A neck chain or leather collar is usually used on dairy goats and they soon become accustomed to being led or restrained by the collar. Collars are useful for securing the goat to a stanchion or wall for such procedures as milking, jugular venipuncture and general examination. Collars can be left on the goat permanently. Neck chains should be made of small, flat links that will not catch easily if the goat rubs against a fence.

Restraint for Dehorning and Castration

Capture the kid, sit down, and fold its legs down into your lap. Place your forearms on its back to keep it from regaining its feet. Grasp the head by positioning your hands on each side of the neck with your fingers wrapped around the mandible (Fig 5). Your thumbs should be placed behind the ears so that after the horns have been removed you can place your thumbs over the wounds to apply pressure.

Restraint for castration is the same as with a lamb.

Restraint for Hoof Trimming

Restraint for trimming the hooves of a goat is much the same as for horses. Have the goat tied or have someone hold the goat using the beard and neck, or by holding the cheeks.

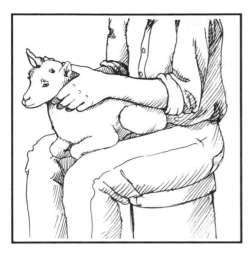

Figure 5. Restraint for dehorning kids.

To trim the front feet, stand slightly in front of the leg on which you will work. Grasp the leg at the ankle, lift and gently bend it at the knee. The foot can be held with one hand while trimming with the other because the hooves on a goat are usually soft enough to be trimmed with shearing scissors. Alternatively, you can place the foot on your bent knee, freeing both hands. Either technique works well.

The rear feet are restrained by standing beside the rear leg on which you will work. Grasp the leg at the ankle, lift and gently stretch it out behind the goat. Rest the outstretched leg on your bent knee or some object high enough so the leg is supported comfortably for the goat.

Restraint for Venipuncture

The cephalic veins of goats are much like those of dogs, and the restraint technique used is similar to that used for dogs (see Chapter 4). Back the goat into a corner and push it sideways against the wall. Place one arm around the goat's neck to stabilize the head and body, and with the other hand grasp the front leg to be used. Wrap your thumb across the top of the leg and roll the vein out to the top of the leg. The venipuncturist must hold the lower (distal) portion of the leg while withdrawing the blood sample.

The cheek hold works well for jugular venipuncture (see Restraint of the Head).

References

1. Edwards LM: Behavior and diseases of the dairy goat. *Veterinary Technician* 4:294-300, 1983.

2. Fowler ME: *Restraint and Handling of Wild and Domestic Animals.* Iowa State Univ Press, Ames, 1978. pp 135-138.

3. Leahy JR and Barrow P: *Restraint of Animals.* Cornell Campus Store, Ithaca, NY, 1953. pp 237-244.

4. Neil DH and Kese ML, in McCurnin DM: *Clinical Textbook for Veterinary Technicians.* Saunders, Philadelphia, 1985. pp 18-19.

10

Restraint of Rodents, Rabbits and Ferrets

Many people have an aversion to handling gerbils, guinea pigs, hamsters, mice, rabbits, rats and ferrets. If they are handled firmly but gently, the chances of being bitten or scratched are small.

Such procedures as giving injections, examination and gastric lavage (gavage) are usually carried out with the animal held in your hand. Other techniques, such as cardiac puncture and orbital sinus venipuncture, require general anesthesia. Rubber-tipped forceps are used to transfer rodents from one cage to another if they cannot be touched because of experimental purposes.

Restraint of Gerbils

The Mongolian gerbil is inquisitive and rapidly becomes tame if handled frequently and gently. They can be aggressive and stomp their hind feet if provoked.

If complete restraint is not necessary, you can pick a gerbil up by scooping it into your hands (Fig 1). Be ready to catch the animal, as they are good jumpers and may jump out of this hold.

Gerbils can also be picked up by their tail (Fig 2). However, be sure to grasp the base of the tail to prevent pulling the skin

Figure 1. Gerbils and hamsters can be picked up by scooping them up in your hands.

Figure 2. Picking up a gerbil by the tail. Grasp the base of the tail to prevent pulling the skin from the tail.

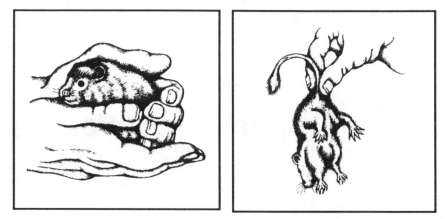

off. This tail hold should only be used to transfer the gerbil from one cage to another, or as the first step in placing them in a more restrictive hold for vaccination and gavage. After grasping the tail, place the gerbil's front feet onto a wire mesh so it can hold onto it. Then grasp the loose skin on the scruff of the neck. Hold the tail, and a back leg if necessary, between your third and fourth finger (Fig 8).

Restraint of Guinea Pigs

Guinea pigs are generally the most docile of all pocket pets. They rarely bite, and only scratch when they are trying to escape capture. Guinea pigs are easily handled because of their docile nature.

To pick a guinea pig up, grasp them over the shoulders and wrap your fingers around the chest. Once the animal is caught, lift it and quickly place your other hand under the rump to support the spine (Fig 3). This is very important for larger guinea pigs and pregnant sows. Be careful not to squeeze the chest area too tightly, as you can impair breathing or damage the ribs. If the underside must be examined or treated, place the animal upside down (belly up) on your forearm (Fig 4).

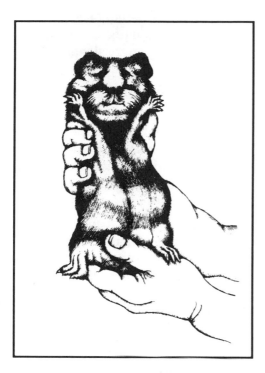

Figure 3. Proper way to lift and carry a guinea pig. Notice the left hand supporting the rear end.

Restraint of Hamsters

Hamsters should be handled frequently to keep them tame. Hamsters show aggression by rolling onto their backs with teeth flashing or by chattering and screaming as you reach into the cage.

Figure 4. Immobilizing a guinea pig by placing its back along the forearm.

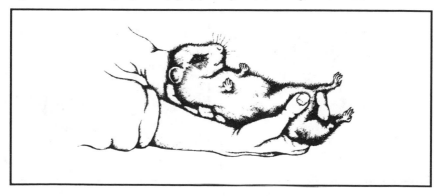

Because of their nocturnal nature, they usually sleep during the day. If you must handle a hamster during the day, it is wise to knock on the cage before reaching in. A sleeping hamster can bite if suddenly awakened.

Never offer your finger for a hamster to sniff, as they usually bite it.

Hamsters have cheek pouches that reach to their shoulders. It is difficult to hold the animal by the scruff of the neck if the pouches are full (Fig 5). When restraining a hamster by the scruff, be sure to grasp as much skin as possible between your fingers so the animal cannot turn and bite you.

Another method of picking up and holding a hamster is to place your palm down over the hamster, wrapping your fingers around its entire body. The head should be pointing toward your wrist (Fig 6). This allows you to easily turn the hamster on its back. Another way to pick up a hamster or to separate fighting hamsters is with a can. A hamster will usually crawl into a can placed in front of it. Hamsters can also be scooped up like gerbils.

Restraint of Mice

Mice tend to unnerve people because they can be skittery and chirp when frightened. They bite only if handled roughly.

Figure 5. Grasp as much of the loose skin as possible on the scruff of a hamster or it can turn and bite.

Figure 6. Restraining a hamster.

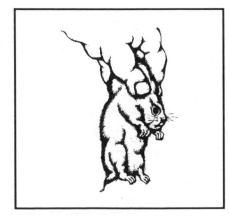
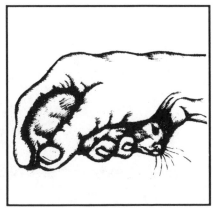

Figure 7. Placing a mouse on a wire grid or mesh keeps it occupied to allow you to grasp the scruff of the neck for a more restrictive hold.

Figure 8. Restraint of a mouse for injections and gavage.

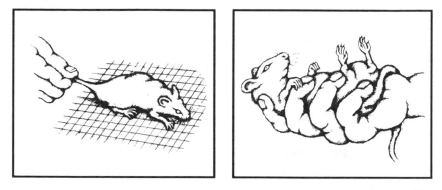

To pick up a mouse, grasp it by the tail. Lift it and quickly place its front feet onto a wire mesh or rough surface, and pull backward gently (Fig 7). This keeps the mouse occupied long enough to grasp the loose skin behind the ears. Then lift the animal, turn your hand over and pin the tail between your little finger and palm (Fig 8). Holding a mouse too tightly may impair its breathing and it can turn blue. However, do not loosen your hold too much, as it may turn and bite. This hold can be used for injections and examination.

If you must hold a mouse by the tail for a longer period, gently bounce or jiggle the mouse to keep it off balance. Be careful not to stop this gentle bouncing, as the mouse can turn and bite.

Restraint chambers can also be used for restraining mice. These have openings for the tail and small holes that can be used to give injections. The disadvantage of a restraint chamber is that it is hard to get a mouse into it. Also, the mouse can turn around in the chamber.

A syringe case with a slit cut on one side of it makes a useful restraint chamber. To place a mouse into this homemade restraint chamber, grasp the tail and gently pull the animal into the syringe case. Place the cap back on the syringe case to stop forward motion. The tail protrudes through the slit for injections.

Restraint of Rats

Rats are intelligent animals that are easily tamed. Two common strains of white rats are the Sprague-Dawley and the Wistar-Lewis, both of which are easily handled. Hooded or Long-Evans rats are black and white or brown and white, and are usually more aggressive than white rats but not as aggressive as the Fischer strain of rats. Rats commonly squeal when lifted or first captured, and bite if provoked.

You must be confident and firm when approaching a rat. Hesitation usually results in a bite. To pick up a rat, place one hand around the chest, wrapping your thumb and index finger around the neck and under the chin (Fig 9). The thumb and index finger are the keys to a successful hold on a rat. Tightening the fingers around the chest only causes the rat to struggle because its breathing is impaired. The animal may faint from lack of oxygen.

Young rats can be lifted by the base of the tail. However, rough handling can tear the skin from the tail, necessitating tail amputation.

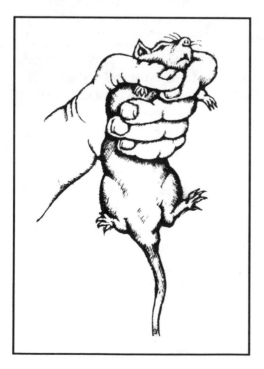

Figure 9. Restraint hold commonly used on rats.

Restraint of Rabbits

Rabbits range in size from 2 to 20 lb. Some aggressive rabbits stomp their feet and rush at the cage door when you open it. Some may even growl. To handle these aggressive rabbits, wear gloves and use a towel or blanket that can be thrown over their bodies until you gain a better hold.

Rabbits should never be lifted by their ears. Picking a rabbit up and carrying it by the ears can cause serious injury to the animal. The correct way to lift a full-grown rabbit is to grasp the scruff of the neck and lift it quickly, supporting the rabbit's rump with your other hand (Fig 10). An immature rabbit can be picked up and carried by grasping the skin over the back and gently lifting. In both cases, *be sure to point the feet of the rabbit away from your body*. Rabbits rarely bite, but they have sharp toenails that can injure you.

Picking a rabbit up by any other method causes it to kick out with its back feet. This may injure its neck muscles and ears if you are holding them, or could break the rabbit's back.

Both young and full-grown rabbits should be carried with their head tucked into the crook of your elbow, their body resting on your forearm and the other hand holding the scruff of the neck (Fig 11). This is comfortable for the rabbit and they seldom resist being held in this manner.

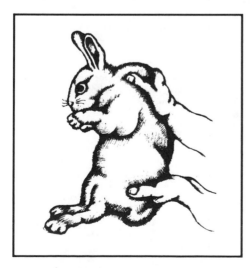

Figure 10. Picking up and carrying a rabbit.

When restraining a rabbit on an examination table, place a towel or mat on the table before placing the animal on it. A smooth surface makes rabbits very nervous, causing them to scramble around in an effort to find stable footing. This can result in injury to you or the rabbit.

One method of examining the underside of a rabbit is to grasp the scruff of the neck in one hand and the back legs in the other, stretching the animal along your forearm. An alternative method is to hold the rabbit by the scruff of the neck with its back against your body. Gently stroke the rabbit's stomach to make it relax and hang limp.

Hypnosis is another method used to have a rabbit lie still on its back. To "hypnotize" a rabbit, grasp the mandible with one hand and the rear legs with the other, and stretch the rabbit out on top of a table. Gently tilt the head back until the rabbit suddenly relaxes. Then maintain a gentle pressure on the head to maintain the "hypnosis." An anxious rabbit can be mesmerized while on its feet by covering the eyes with your hand and applying gentle pressure to its temples.

A restraint technique that works well for intramuscular injections is to hold the rabbit by the scruff of the neck with one hand and support the back with the other. Set the rabbit's rear on the table and lean its back against your body. The per-

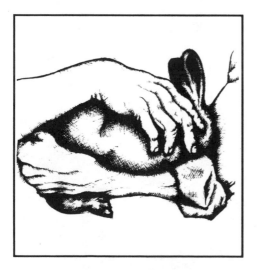

Figure 11. Proper hold for carrying rabbits for longer distances.

son giving the injection can then grasp a hind leg and give the injection (Fig 12).

Restraint devices commonly used on rabbits include towels, bleeding boxes and rabbit boards. A towel wrapped tightly around the rabbit's body has a calming effect and prevents the rabbit from scratching with its feet. A bleeding box is a small box that holds the rabbit's body and has a space for the ears to be extracted or the entire head to protrude. A rabbit board looks much like the trough used on pigs except that it is smaller (see Chapter 7). The feet are tied as with pigs, but the rabbit is anesthetized or "hypnotized" before being placed into the trough.

After the examination or treatment is completed, return the animal to its cage by placing its rear legs down first and retaining your hold on the scruff of the neck. This is necessary because rabbits typically try to jump away when their rear feet touch the ground. If the rabbit is pointed toward a wall, it may jump into the wall and injure itself. Retain your hold on the scruff of the neck until the animal has calmed before releasing it.

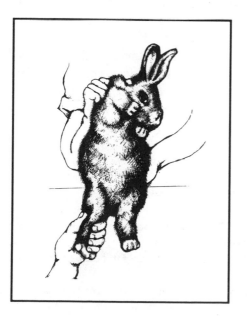

Figure 12. Restraint of a rabbit for intramuscular injection.

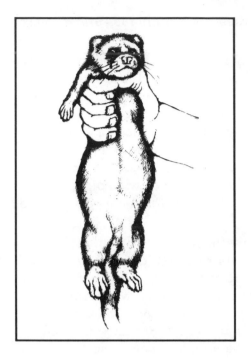

Figure 13. Carrying an uncooperative ferret.

Restraint of Ferrets

Most ferrets are easy to hold. They are easily tamed and rarely bite. However, females with young should be respected because they are quite protective. A difficult ferret can be handled like a rat, with the hand over its shoulder and the fingers wrapped around its chest (Fig 13). They quickly release their grip if they do bite. If they do not release their grip, dunking them in water or placing them under a running faucet causes them to let go.

References

1. Brunckhorst B: *Handling, Restraint and Gavage of the Rabbit.* Prentice Hall, Tarrytown, NY.

2. Harkness JE and Wagner JE: *The Biology and Medicine of Rabbits and Rodents.* Lea & Febiger, Philadelphia, 1989.

3. Hafez E: *Reproduction and Breeding Techniques for Laboratory Animals.* Lea & Febiger, Philadelphia, 1970.

4. Sirois M: *The Pet Guinea Pig.* American Assn Lab Animal Science, Joliet, IL, 1984.

5. Vickery B: *Handling, Restraint and Gavage of the Hamster & Gerbil.* Prentice Hall, Tarrytown, NY.

6. Rooks WH *et al*: *Handling, Restraint and Gavage of the Rat.* Prentice Hall, Tarrytown, NY.

7. Williams K: *Practical Guide to Laboratory Animals.* Mosby, St. Louis, 1976.

11

Restraint of Birds

Caged birds, such as parakeets (budgerigars), canaries, finches, parrots, cockatiels, mynahs and lories, are being seen more in veterinary practice than ever before. Clients have found these pets to be perfect for apartment living, and these birds fit well into an owner's active lifestyle.

Birds are highly sensitive to stress, and rough handling can cause broken wings or legs, progression of a disease process and even death. But birds can defend themselves with their beaks. They also have very sharp toenails, and larger birds can injure you with their wings. It takes practice and patience to work with these animals successfully and safely. As with other species, you must be patient and even-tempered, using the least restraint necessary to get the job done.

Transport to the Clinic

Advise the client to bring the bird in its own cage after removing all toys, emptying the water dish and removing all but one perch. This lessens the chance of accidental injury in transit. The food dish and the droppings tray should remain in the cage so they can be evaluated at the clinic. If the weather is cold, the car should be warmed and a blanket placed over the entire cage. This helps prevent hypothermia and helps the bird feel secure. During hot weather, be sure the bird is not in

the path of the air conditioner vents, as sick birds do not tolerate drafts well.

In the examination room, have the client remove the re-
maining perch, food and water dish. This makes the job of capturing the bird a lot easier, and prevents injury to the bird.

Capturing the Bird

Most tame birds have been trained to hop onto your finger
or wrist, after which you can easily grasp them from behind. If
the bird is small to medium sized, lay its back into your palm
and use your index finger and thumb to steady the head. For
larger birds, use one hand to steady the head and the other to
hold the wings and legs. With tame birds, the owner may be
the best one to hold them because the bird may then feel more
secure. If the bird must be transferred from the owner to you,
secure the head first, then the wings.

Small to medium-sized birds can be caught with one hand
by approaching them from the back and quickly but firmly
grasping them with index finger and thumb placed on either
side of the head. The other fingers encircle the thorax and the
little finger encircles the legs (Fig 1). Be careful not to exert

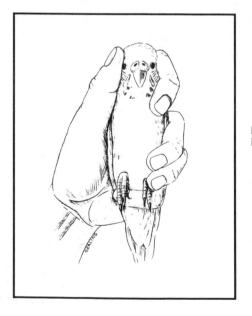

Figure 1. Finger position for restraining a small to medium-sized bird.

too much pressure on the thorax, as you may cause the bird to suffocate. If necessary, you can wear light leather gloves to protect yourself from bites.

Large birds must be caught with 2 hands. Approach from the back, with one hand grasping the back of the head first and then quickly securing the wings with the other (Fig 2). Heavy leather gloves should be worn when handling these birds because they can crush fingers or inflict severe wounds with their beaks. After the bird is captured, remove the gloves, one hand at a time, as they reduce your tactile awareness and may reduce your awareness of how tightly you are holding the bird.

If a bird is very antagonistic, you can divert its attention with a glove or towel. While the bird is biting that, quickly grasp the bird as described above. Turning out or dimming the lights helps calm nervous birds so they do not flutter around in the cage, possibly injuring themselves. Also, birds can become hyperthermic quite rapidly in their attempts to escape.

A light hand towel can also be used to capture a caged bird. Once covered, the bird usually holds still so you can grasp it

Figure 2. Restraint of a large bird, using 2 hands and heavy protective gloves.

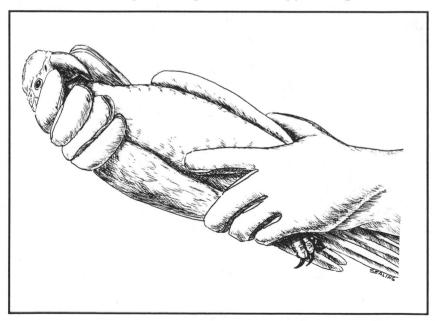

with your hands. A disadvantage is that you never know quite where you are grasping the bird, so you could injure it or it may have the opportunity to bite you. Once you have the bird, it can be difficult to uncover the right area for examination without releasing the bird.

If you must capture a bird in a large aviary, a net is necessary. Once the bird is in the net, quickly pin the wings close to the body and restrain the head so the bird does not injure itself or you.

Restraint for Medical Procedures

Oral Medication

Liquid oral medication is given with the bird's head elevated above the horizontal plane to prevent aspiration. Hold the head and body as described before for capturing the bird (Figs 1, 2). If a tube is to be passed into the stomach, the beak must be held open so the bird does not bite through the tube.

A paper clip works well as a speculum for small to medium-sized birds, but manufactured specula should be used for large birds. To apply the paper clip speculum, tilt the bird slightly to one side and place the upper beak in the short inside loop of the clip. Then swing the clip down and place the end inside the lower beak (Fig 3).

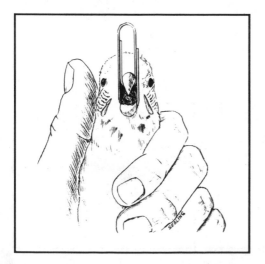

Figure 3. Use of paper clip as an oral speculum.

Injections

Injections can be given by subcutaneous (SC) or intramuscular (IM) routes. To give a SC injection, hold the bird's head with thumb and index finger, and support the wings and legs with other fingers for small to medium-sized birds, or with the other hand for large birds. Slowly stretch one wing out so the injection can be given in the axillary region (Fig 4). For IM injection, hold the bird in the same way but present the pectoral or quadriceps muscle to the person giving the injection.

Venipuncture

Venipuncture can be done on the right jugular vein or the brachial vein located in the wing. For jugular venipuncture, hold the bird so its breast rests against the palm of your hand. The head is held between the index and middle fingers, and should be turned to the left and slightly extended. The thumb is used to hold back the feathers and occlude the jugular vein (Fig 5). Note that extending the head too far to the side can kink the trachea, causing the bird to suffocate. The brachial vein can be exposed using the same hold as for SC injection (Fig 4).

Ocular Medication

The eyes are medicated by holding the bird as described for injections, except the eye being medicated is turned upward (Fig 4).

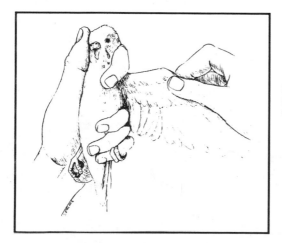

Figure 4. Restraint for subcutaneous injections and brachial venipuncture.

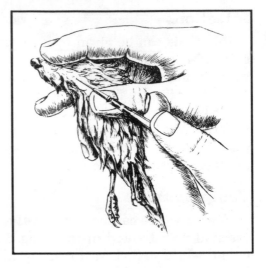

Figure 5. Restraint for jugular venipuncture.

Splint Application

Fractured wings and legs are often treated by application of tape splints. To restrain a bird for splint application, hold the bird in one hand with the head held between index finger and thumb. Gently turn the bird so it is in dorsal recumbency and very gently grasp the affected leg by the toes (Fig 6). Follow the doctor's instructions on how far to straighten the leg.

Figure 6. Restraint for application of a leg splint.

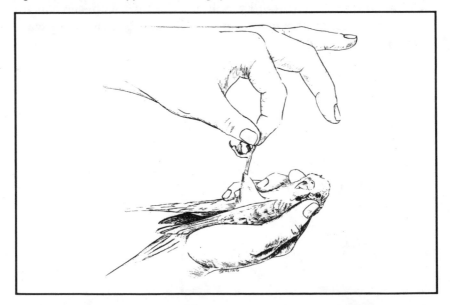

For application of a wing splint, the bird is held in an upright position, with one hand steadying the head and the other hand holding the legs, tail and tips of the wings. The bird should be held facing the doctor and held up so that you and the doctor are not bent over.

Radiography

In restraining birds for radiographic procedures, small to medium-sized birds can be taped directly to the cassette with paper tape and weighed down with lead-lined gloves. Large birds usually must be held using your hands protected by lead-lined gloves. Remember that your hands and fingers should *never* be in the primary beam. Tape, gauze bandages, radiographic weights and/or anesthesia should be used as needed to hold the bird in position.

Elizabethan Collar

An Elizabethan collar is often necessary to prevent a bird from picking at its bandages or a wound. Various materials can be used to fashion collars for these animals, including playing cards, plastic detergent bottles, pieces of cardboard and pieces of x-ray film for small to medium-sized birds. Larger birds require heavier material, such as thick leather or very sturdy plastic.

Beak Restraint

If the bird is a ferocious biter, you can tape the beak shut. If the beak is long and pointed, you can place a cork on the end of it. Be careful when removing the tape from the beak, as the bird may try to retaliate by biting.

References

Burr: *Companion Bird Medicine.* Iowa State Univ Press, Ames, 1987. pp 20-27.

Fowler: *Restraint and Handling of Wild and Domestic Animals.* Iowa State Univ Press, Ames, 1978. pp 262-285.

Petrak: *Diseases of Cage and Aviary Birds.* 2nd ed. Lea & Febiger, Philadelphia, 1982. pp 229-230, 258-268, 389-392.

Steiner and Davis: *Caged Bird Medicine.* Iowa State Univ Press, Ames, 1981.

Appendix 1

Gender Names

Dogs

Male: dog
Female: bitch
Newborn/young: pup

Cats

Male: tom
Female: queen
Newborn/young: kitten

Horses

Male: stallion or stud
Female: mare
Young male: colt
Young female: filly
Newborn (either sex): foal
Castrated male: gelding

Cattle

Male: bull
Female: cow
Young male: bullock, bull calf
Young female: heifer
Newborn: calf
Castrated male: steer

Pigs

Male: boar
Female: sow

Male castrated after maturity: barrow
Male castrated before maturity: stag
Young female: gilt
Young of either sex: shoat
Newborn: piglet

Sheep

Male: ram or buck
Female: ewe
Newborn/young: lamb
Castrated male: wether

Goats

Male: billy or buck
Female: nanny or doe
Newborn/young: kid
Castrated male: chevon

Rabbits

Male: buck
Female: doe
Newborn/young: kindling

Ferrets

Male: hob
Female: jill
Newborn/young: kit

Appendix 2

Physiologic Data

Species	Rectal Temperature	Pulse Rate (/min)	Respiratory Rate (/min)
Dogs	100.5-102.5	70-180	10-30
Cats	100.5-102.5	110-130	20-30
Horses	99.5-101.3	28-50	8-16
Cattle	100.5-103	40-70	10-30
Pigs	100-104	58-100	8-18
Sheep	102-104	60-90	12-19
Goats	102-104	60-90	12-19
Rabbits	99.1-102.9	250-300	—
Ferrets	100-104.1	216-242	—
Mice	95-102.6	—	—
Guinea Pigs	99.3-103	230-300	—
Rats	96.8-102.1	250-500	—
Hamsters	97-102.3	275-425	—
Gerbils	96.3-102.8	—	—

Appendix 3

Glossary

Aggressive: a fighting disposition.

Anesthesia: loss of sensation with or without loss of consciousness.

Bight: a sharp bend in a rope.

Bolus: medication delivered in one large dose or a preparation of oral medication given to large animals.

Bovine: of or relating to oxen or cattle.

Brachycephalic: referring to short-nosed breeds of dogs, such as the Boxer, English Bulldog and Pug.

Butt: to thrust or push with the head or horns.

Calving: the act of a cow's giving birth.

Canine: of or relating to dogs.

Caprine: of or relating to goats.

Cast: to throw to the ground, usually with a variety of ropes and knots.

Caudal: situated in or directed toward the hind part of the body.

Cephalic vein: a blood vessel located in the cranial aspect of the front leg.

Cervical vertebrae: spinal bones in the neck.

Chute: a capture device made of metal or wood that restrains cattle.

Coccygeal vertebrae: spinal bones of the tail.

Commissure: junction between 2 parts, such as the lips or eyelids.

Constructive tonalities: using the voice in a commanding way.

Corral: pen or enclosure for confining or capturing livestock.

Cranial: situated in or directed toward the front part of the body.

Distal: away from the point of attachment or axis of the body.

Distraction technique: using mild pain to distract the attention of an animal so a procedure can be performed.

Dock: the part of an animal's tail left after amputation.

Dorsal: toward the spine or upper side of the body.

Drench: large dose of medicine mixed with liquid and given down the throat of an animal.

End: end of a rope that can be freely moved about.

Far side: the right side of a horse.

Farrow: the act of a sow's giving birth.

Feline: of or relating to cats.

Femoral vein: located on the medial side of the hind leg, between the sartorius and gracilis muscles.

Fetlock: leg joint above the hoof of a horse or other hooved animal.

Flank: laying an animal on its side.

Foaling: the act of a mare's giving birth.

Friable: easily broken or pulverized.

Gauntlets: heavy leather gloves used to restrain animals.

Gurney: a wheeled cot or stretcher.

Half hitch: complete circle formed in a rope when making a knot or hitch.

Head shy: wariness of having the head approached or touched.

Hematoma: swelling or mass of blood confined to an organ, tissue or space, caused by a break in a blood vessel.

Herbivore: plant-eating animal.

Hitch: temporary fastening of a rope to a hook, post or other object with the rope arranged so the standing part forces the end against the object with sufficient pressure to prevent slipping.

Hobbles: device used to fasten together the legs of an animal to prevent straying.

Hock: the tarsal joint or region in the hind limb of animals that corresponds to the ankle in people.

Hurdle: portable panel used to herd livestock.

Hyperthermia: abnormally high body temperature.

Hypothermia: abnormally low body temperature.

Hypoxia: deficiency of oxygen reaching the tissues of the body.

Jugular veins: paired major blood vessels running lateral to the trachea.

Kindling: the act of a female rabbit's giving birth.

Knot: intertwining of 1 or 2 ropes in which the pressure of the standing part of the rope alone prevents the end from slipping.

Lambing: the act of a ewe's giving birth.

Lateral: situated in or directed toward the side of the body, away from the body axis.

Lateral recumbency: reclining on the side of the body.

Lateral saphenous vein: blood vessel on the lateral aspect of the leg just distal to the hock.

Lavage: washing out of a cavity.

Lumbar vertebrae: spinal bones between the chest and pelvis.

Mandible: lower jaw.

Medial: situated in or directed toward the axis of the body.

Metatarsus: part of the hind foot in quadrupeds, distal to the tarsus or ankle.

Muzzle: covering for an animal's mouth to prevent eating or biting.

Near side: the left side of a horse.

Obese: excessively fat.

Occluding: close or hold off, such as occluding a vessel for venipuncture.

Overhand knot: basic knot used in more complex knots.

Ovine: of or relating to sheep.

Palpation: to examine by touch.

Per os: by mouth.

Pinch biting: biting with the incisors of a muzzled dog or cat.

Pinna: ear flap.

Porcine: of or relating to pigs.

Proximal: toward the point of attachment or axis of the body.

Queening: the act of a female cat's giving birth.

Restraint: forcefully preventing movement or activity by physical or chemical means.

Stanchion: device that fits loosely around a cow's neck and limits forward and backward motion.

Standing part: longer end of the rope that is attached to the animal.

Stocks: small square restraining pen with a front and back gate.

Territory: area, such as a nesting or denning site and foraging range, defended by an animal or group of animals.

Thoracic vertebrae: spinal bones of the chest area.

Throw: the wrapping of one rope around another to make a knot.

Twitch: chain, rope or strap that is tightened over a horse's lip as a restraining device.

Venipuncture: puncture of a vein for withdrawal of blood or injection.

Venipuncturist: one who performs a venipuncture.

Ventral: away from the spine or upper side of the body.

Whelping: the act of a bitch's giving birth.

Withers: the area between the shoulder blades of a horse.

Index

A

adhesive tape, 38, 62

B

birds, 131-137
    beak, 137
    capture, 132-134
    Elizabethan collar, 137
    eye, 135
    injections, 135
    medicating, 134, 135
    radiography, 137
    splint application, 136
    transport, 131
    venipuncture, 135
blindfold, horses, 79
bowline, 19, 20
bowline on bight, 20, 21

C

calves, 93, 94
capture pole, 48
casting, horses, 81
    pigs, 102-105
cats, 25-40
    adhesive tape, 38
    distraction techniques, 27
    examination, 33
    fetal hold, 27
    friendly cats, 28
    head, 26
    injections, 34-36
    leather gloves, 29
    legs, 26
    medicating, 33, 34
    muzzles, 39
    New York hold, 35
    precautions, 26
    pretzel hold, 38
    restraint bag, 32, 37
    scrunch technique, 33
    towels, 36
    unfriendly cats, 29
    venipuncture, 30-32
cattle, 85-95
    calves, 93, 94
    chutes, 86, 87
    flank rope, 93
    flanking, 94
    halter, 88
    head, 87-90
    herding, 85, 86
    hobbles, 92
    legs, 92, 93
    mouth speculum, 89
    nose lead, 89
    nose ring, 90
    tail jacking, 91
    tail tying, 92
chain shank, 75-77
chutes, 86, 87
clove hitch, 21
cradle, 79
cross tying, horses, 77

D

dental procedures, horses, 77
distraction techniques, cats, 27
dogs, 41-63
    aggressive dogs, 44, 51
    caged dogs, 50-52
    capture pole, 48
    carrying, 52
    Elizabethan collar, 61
    examination, 53-55
    hobbles, 62